Parenting a Child with Attention-Deficit/Hyperactivity Disorder

Parenting a Child with Attention-Deficit/ Hyperactivity Disorder

Jane N. Hannah

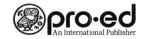
pro·ed
An International Publisher

8700 Shoal Creek Boulevard
Austin, Texas 78757-6897
1-800-897-3202 Fax 1-800-397-7633
order online at http://www.proedinc.com

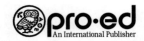

© 1999 by PRO-ED, Inc.
8700 Shoal Creek Boulevard
Austin, Texas 78757-6897
1-800-897-3202 Fax 1-800-397-7633
order online at http://www.proedinc.com

Library of Congress Cataloging-in-Publication Data
Hannah, Jane.
    Parenting a child with attention-deficit/hyperactivity disorder
/ Jane N. Hannah.
      p.   cm.
    Includes bibliographical references.
    ISBN 0-89079-791-9 (alk. paper)
    1. Attention-deficit hyperactivity disorder.   2. Hyperactive
children—Behavior modification.   I. Title.
RJ506.K9 H37   1999
618.92'8589—dc21

                        98-27891
                          CIP

This book is designed in Goudy.

Production Director: Alan Grimes
Production Coordinator: Dolly Fisk Jackson
Managing Editor: Chris Olson
Art Director: Thomas Barkley
Designer: Jason Crosier
Staff Copyeditor: Martin Wilson
Reprints Buyer: Alicia Woods
Preproduction Coordinator: Chris Anne Worsham
Project Editor: Teri Sperry
Publishing Assistant: John Means Cooper

Printed in the United States of America

1 2 3 4 5 6 7 8 9 10   03 02 01 00 99

Contents

Preface

In my work with parents over the last 27 years, I have found that they are searching for practical answers to their parenting problems, especially if those parents have children with special needs. This fact became personal after having my second child. My first child, Julie, was a baby with an "easy" temperament. Because she was so easy to parent, it was difficult for me to empathize with parents who were experiencing significant problems with their children. I was quick to assume that parents who were experiencing difficulty in their parenting must be doing something wrong. It was not until I had my second child, Thomas, that I realized that some children were temperamentally different. I tried my same limited parenting strategies with Thomas, but he continued to push the limits. He tested my authority in almost every incidence. At first, I thought it was because his father and I were divorced and that the underlying issues related to the loss of his father were the cause for his problems. Later, my new suspicions were confirmed, and it was determined that Thomas had a learning disability and an attention-deficit/hyperactivity disorder (ADHD).

As I discovered with Julie, as well as with my third child, Emily, I really didn't need an arsenal of parenting strategies to be a "good parent." Julie and Emily made me look like a "super parent." But I found with Thomas, as many parents find, that my self-esteem as a parent was highly dependent on how well he behaved and stayed out of trouble. I knew that I needed to learn all I could about his disorders and how to help him reach adulthood successfully. Being a special education teacher, I had some training in behavioral analysis; however, even with this knowledge, parenting was never easy where Thomas was concerned.

As my journey progressed in my training and experience, I began sharing the mistakes and successes with other parents who found themselves in the same parenting dilemmas. In 1991 Vanderbilt Medical Center began a treatment program for children with ADHD. As director of this program, I worked directly with the children as well as their parents to address the problems created by this condition. I soon learned that parents were thirsty for practical ways to address their children's problems. They did not want a theoretical or research approach, but rather "down-to-earth" suggestions. I also quickly learned that many of the parents with whom I worked exhibited some of the same characteristics as their children. As I discussed topics each week in our parenting classes, I observed that many parents experienced difficulty with the organization of my handouts and follow-through with the assignments. Thus, prior to the 1995 Summer Treatment Program, I compiled all the information into a parenting guide for these families. The parents no longer needed to keep up with all the materials I was giving them.

This book has evolved since 1995 into its current status as I have received input and advice from parents of children with ADHD. While the information presented in this book is based on sound research in what we have found to work with the child with ADHD, I have attempted to share this information using a concrete, practical-advice approach. The personal examples in the book are real; only the names have been changed to protect the parents and their children. I have attempted to address as many of the parenting concerns as possible in this book, but each year parents have presented me with new problems that needed immediate attention and that I was unable to address in only 8 weeks of training. Thus, I have included in Chapter 9 questions that have been asked by our parents and possible solutions. I have found that when parents are serious about their parenting but open minded enough to try different approaches to solving problems, a greater degree of success can be realized. It does not mean that all the problems will disappear, nor that parenting is made easy. Parenting is very difficult, especially with children who are strong willed and who demonstrate a high rate of acting-out behaviors. While this book is written specifically for the parent of a child with ADHD, the principles underlying the advice are just "good, sound parenting" techniques. What will work for the child with ADHD will work for his or her siblings.

This book is written for parents seeking help in their parenting, and the Appendixes contain suggestions for mental health professionals who may desire to lead parenting groups using this book as a study guide. This book will be primarily useful to the parent of a child who is approximately 5 to 11 years of age. There is, however, additional information in Chapter 10 that addresses some of the issues for the child making the transition into adolescence. While the information in this book can be valuable to parents, it does have its limitations. You are encouraged to identify a professional who can assist you in dealing with problems that are more serious or issues for which you feel you need expert advice.

Finally, I would like to acknowledge the encouragement and support provided by numerous individuals in the preparation of this book. First, without the experience of living with and loving a child, an adolescent, and an adult with ADHD, I could not have fully understood the magnitude of the need for such a book. Thus, I thank Thomas for the inspiration to write this book. I also want to thank Julie and Emily for their support and "on-the-job" training they have given me. Emily, Thomas, and Julie have been the recipients of my parenting successes as well as my parenting mistakes. Hopefully, the parents who read this book will obtain helpful advice from my experiences.

In addition, without the support, encouragement, and suggestions of many of the parents who have participated in the parent training classes, this book would not be possible. My sincere gratitude is given to Barbie Baker for the countless examples she has provided me of living with an adolescent with ADHD and for proofing the manuscript. I thank my stepchildren, Dolly and Mancy, for their sense of humor in learning to enjoy Thomas's excursions. A special thanks is given to my parents, Louise and Olen Norris, who provided support and encouragement in my own parenting. Lastly, my gratitude and sincere appreciation are given to Larry Pendergrass, my husband, who encouraged me, patiently waited for me while I worked on the manuscript, and cooked many meals while I was completing this book as well as while I worked with many of our parents. I sincerely thank each one of you.

If I Had My Child
To Raise Over Again

If I had my child to raise all over again,
I'd build self-esteem first, and the house later.
I'd finger-paint more, and point the finger less.
I would do less correcting and more connecting.
I'd take my eyes off my watch, and watch with my eyes.

I would care to know less and know to care more.
I'd take more hikes and fly more kites.
I'd stop playing serious, and seriously play.
I would run through more fields and gaze at more stars.

I'd do more hugging and less tugging.
I'd see the oak tree in the acorn more often.
I would be firm less often, and affirm much more.
I'd model less about the love of power,
And more about the power of love.

By Diane Loomans

Note. From *Full Esteem Ahead* (p. 194), by D. Loomans with J. Loomans, 1994, Tiburon, CA: H J Kramer. Copyright 1994 by H J Kramer. Reprinted with permission.

Understanding Attention-Deficit/ Hyperactivity Disorder

Matthew's parents came into our office at the request of his pediatrician. Already at the young age of 7 years, he had experienced significant behavioral and social problems. At the age of 4 years, the director of his day-care center reported that he was aggressive and that he was experiencing difficulty following rules and getting along with his peers. At the age of 5, his Sunday School teacher at church told his mother not to bring him back until his behavior was better. When he was in the first grade, his behavior became increasingly worse. Matthew's first-grade instruction was in an open classroom, with his class sharing a large pod with three others. In this setting, Matthew was aggressive to his peers, both verbally and physically; he experienced significant difficulty completing his assignments and turning them in; and he was in constant motion. His teacher reported that when other children were not near him, he was rather easy to manage and was more in control of his behavior, but when he was in a group of more than three children, he was extremely disruptive. At the time we first saw him, he said that he thought he was "stupid" and that no one liked him.

In order to determine the reasons for Matthew's behavioral and social problems, his parents and teachers were asked to complete several checklists and information forms. This information was helpful in determining the extent of Matthew's difficulties in the home setting as well as in the school environment. Review of this information revealed that Matthew was experiencing the following problems: overactivity, excessive talking, impulsive responding, failing to complete assignments, difficulty following oral directions, negative peer interactions, and underachievement in written assignments and in phonics. After a review of this information, Matthew was scheduled for a team evaluation conducted by a clinical psychologist, educational specialist, language pathologist, developmental pediatrician, and clinical social worker. This evaluation was suggested because Matthew was experiencing not only behavioral problems but also academic problems. Thus, it was necessary to determine whether Matthew's problems were the result of a learning disability, language disorder, or ADHD.

❓ What is Attention-Deficit/Hyperactivity Disorder (ADHD)?

ADHD is a neurodevelopmental disorder (sometimes referred to as a behavioral disorder) with a persistent pattern of inattention and/or hyperactivity and/or impulsivity that is more frequent and severe than is typically observed in individuals at a comparable level of development. While ADHD is thought to be associated with a disturbance in functioning of neurotransmitters in the brain (Jensen and Garfinkel, 1988), the disorder is defined not by its cause but rather by the three primary clinical symptoms:

- inattention
- hyperactivity
- impulsivity

1

According to the *Diagnostic and Statistical Manual of Mental Disorders* (DSM-IV; American Psychiatric Association, 1994), there are three subtypes of ADHD. These are based on two dimensions. These are as follows:

- ADHD, Predominantly Inattentive Type
- ADHD, Predominantly Hyperactive-Impulsive Type
- ADHD, Combined Type (meeting criteria for both dimensions)

In the *Inattentive* dimension, the individual must exhibit 6 of 9 of the following behaviors to a marked degree (rated as "often" occurrences):

- makes careless mistakes

- has difficulty sustaining attention in tasks

- seems not to listen when spoken to directly

- does not follow through on instructions or fails to finish tasks

- has difficulty organizing tasks

- avoids, dislikes, or is reluctant to engage in tasks requiring sustained mental attention

- loses things necessary for tasks

- is easily distracted

- is forgetful in daily activities

In the *Hyperactive-Impulsive* dimension, the individual must exhibit at least 6 of 9 of the following behaviors (rated as "often" occurrences):

- often fidgets with hands or feet or squirms in seat
- is unable to remain seated when expected to do so
- moves around excessively (is restless) in situations in which it is inappropriate
- has difficulty engaging in leisure activities quietly
- is "on the go" or acts as if "driven by a motor"
- talks excessively
- blurts out answers before questions have been completed
- has difficulty awaiting turn
- interrupts or intrudes on others

In addition, the criteria listed below must be met.

- Some symptoms must be present before the age of 7 years.
- Symptoms must be present for at least 6 months.
- Some impairment from the symptoms must be demonstrated in two or more settings.
- There must be evidence of clinically significant impairment in social, academic, or occupational functioning.
- The symptoms do not occur exclusively during the course of a Pervasive Development Disorder, Schizophrenia, or other Psychotic Disorder, and are not better accounted for by another mental disorder (e.g., Mood Disorder, Anxiety Disorder, Dissociative Disorder, or a Personality Disorder).

? *Do all children with ADHD look alike?*

No, they don't all look like Matthew. Some may exhibit aggressive acts that may even appear planned. Some may be explosive and very impulsive. Others may demonstrate significant peer relationship problems because they appear aloof, and others may have problems with social functioning because they are aggressive or socially clumsy. Some children have academic problems because of inattention or learning problems, and others score high on group achievement tests and appear to know the answer before the teacher asks the question.

? *Is this a new condition?*

No. A German physician, Heinrich Hoffmann, described a hyperactive child as "Fidgety Phil" and an inattentive child as "Harry Look in the Air" in a book he wrote in 1848. From 1940 to 1960 this child was referred to as "Brain-Damaged." In the period between 1960 and 1969, the condition was referred to as "hyperactive child syndrome." By the early 1970s the disorder had broadened to include attention deficits. It was described as attention-deficit disorder in the 1980s and as attention-deficit/hyperactivity disorder in 1987. The new classification system with the three subtypes of ADHD was instituted in 1994 when the DSM-IV was published.

? *How is ADHD diagnosed?*

If you are concerned that your child is demonstrating behaviors that are suggestive of ADHD, first you may want to discuss this with your child's pediatrician. It is always advisable for the pediatrician to complete a thorough physical examination in order to rule out the presence of any medical problems that might be causing these behaviors. Next, consult with your child's teacher or another individual (e.g., day-care worker) who knows your child well. Since the symptoms must be present in two settings, a conversation with his or her teacher, day-care director, or another person who has observed your child in a group setting is an important step in the evaluation process. If your child is demonstrating these symptoms in some form in two settings, and you have ruled out any medical problems, you have several approaches to take in the diagnostic process.

You may ask the public school to complete the assessment. Even if your child does not attend a public school, the school system in which your child is zoned can complete a free evaluation. Most schools usually have a support team that is convened to discuss what should be done to address the teacher's or your concerns. This team may decide that an evaluation appears warranted. While the evaluation is in process, the support team will likely initiate some interventions within the classroom to address your child's specific problems. The school's evaluation process *may* include the following:

- a collection of behavioral data through parent and teacher checklists and by observing your child in his or her regular classroom

- a review of your child's school and social history

- a comprehensive psychoeducational and language assessment to rule out any learning problems that could be causing your child's problems in school. If no learning problems appear to be the reason for the inattention or behavioral or social problems, the psychological, educational, and/or language evaluations may not be needed.

Under the changes in the Individuals with Disabilities Education Act of 1990 (IDEA), the school may now diagnose ADHD, or the school system may send its results to a physician to make the diagnosis. The school system's procedure for diagnosing ADHD should be documented in writing.

Another option for this assessment is to request that the evaluation be completed by a private or university facility. Carefully select this agency by checking with other parents, educators, and your child's pediatrician for a facility that understands the disorder. A reputable agency will collect information related to your child's functioning from two sources and will have experience assessing and working with children and/or adolescents with ADHD. Most private agencies will request that the child's teacher complete checklists and provide the agency with information related to the child's academic, social, and behavioral functioning in the school setting. Often, these professionals will send checklists to the school and will request school records before determining who needs to be on the evaluation team. Specialists who may be a part of the evaluation team include clinical or developmental psychologists, social workers, educational specialists, language pathologists, developmental pediatricians, and child psychiatrists. The evaluation team will complete a medical, family, and social history assessment, a physical examination, an assessment of your child's school functioning in the behavioral, academic, and social domains, and screen for possible emotional problems.

It should be noted that there is no single test that can be used to diagnose ADHD. In order to determine whether a child meets the diagnostic criteria for ADHD, information must be gathered from several sources:

- *Parents:* Information can be obtained by interviewing the parents and by completing behavior rating scales, such as the following:

    Attention-Deficit Disorders Evaluation Scale, Home Version (ADDES). McCarney. Columbia, MO: Hawthorne.

    Attention-Deficit/Hyperactivity Disorder Test (ADHDT). Gilliam. PRO-ED. 8700 Shoal Creek Boulevard, Austin, TX 78757 (512-451-3246).

    The Behavior Assessment System for Children (BASC). Reynolds and Kamphaus. May be ordered from AGS, 4201 Woodland Road, Circle Pines, MN 55014-1796 (800-328-2560).

    Child Behavior Checklist (CBCL). Achenbach. University of Vermont, 1 South Prospect St., Burlington, VT 05401.

    Conners' Parent Rating Scales. Conners. May be ordered through A. D. D. WareHouse (800-233-9273).

- *Older children and adolescents:* Information should be gathered from the older child through interviews and checklists, such as the following:

    Attention-Deficit/Hyperactivity Disorder Test (ADHDT). Gilliam. PRO-ED, 8700 Shoal Creek Boulevard, Austin, TX 78757 (512-451-3246).

    Behavior Assessment System for Children (BASC). Reynolds and Kamphaus. May be ordered from AGS, 4201 Woodland Road, Circle Pines, MN 55014-1796 (800-328-2560).

    Copeland Symptom Checklist for Attention Deficit Disorders—Adolescent Version. Copeland. May be ordered from A. D. D. WareHouse (800-233-9273).

    Youth Self-Report for Ages 11–18. Achenbach. University of Vermont, 1 South Prospect St., Burlington, VT 05401.

- *Teacher:* It is important to obtain information from your child's primary teacher. This information may include subjective information (e.g., classroom observations, interview or referral form with questions related to child's functioning in the classroom), as well as systematic information from norm-referenced checklists. Possible rating scales for teachers include the following:

ADD-H Comprehensive Teacher's Rating Scale (ACTeRS). Ullmann, Sleator, and Sprague. MetriTech, Inc., 111 North Market Street, Champaign, IL. May be ordered from PAR, Inc. (800-331-8373) or A. D. D. WareHouse (800-328-2560)

Attention Deficit Disorders Evaluation Scale—School Version (ADDES-SV). McCarney. Columbia, MO: Hawthorne.

Attention-Deficit Hyperactivity Disorder Test (ADHDT). Gilliam. PRO-ED, 8700 Shoal Creek Boulevard, Austin, Texas 78757 (512-451-3246).

Behavior Assessment System for Children (BASC). Reynolds and Kamphaus. May be ordered from AGS, 4201 Woodland Road, Circle Pines, MN 55014-1796 (800-328-2560).

Conners' Teacher Rating Scale—Revised. Conners. May be ordered through A. D. D. WareHouse (800-233-9273).

Teacher Report Form. Achenbach. University of Vermont, 1 South Prospect St., Burlington, VT 05401.

- *Impairment assessment:* A child with ADHD does not always demonstrate an academic impairment when given individually administered educational tests. If there are no learning problems in addition to the ADHD, the child will typically perform well on these tests. A child can be impaired educationally, however, even though he or she does well in a one-on-one testing setting. Thus, in addition to educational tests, it may be necessary to assess academic impairment in other ways. Before the diagnosis can be made, an impairment must be documented in the social, educational, or occupational setting. Impairment may be established by using the following procedures:

1. Review of past school performance (e.g., school records, information from past and current teachers, history of school suspensions, reports of behavior incidents).

2. Completion of checklists. These may include the following:

AAMR Adaptive Behavior Scales—School, Second Edition (ABS-5:2). Lambert, Leland, and Nihira. May be purchased from The Psychological Corporation, San Antonio, TX (800-211-8378).

Behavior Rating Profile. Brown and Hammill. PRO-ED, Austin, TX (512-451-3246).

Home Situations Questionnaire. Barkley. Guilford Press, New York, NY.

School Situations Questionnaire. Barkley. Guilford Press, New York, NY.

? What other conditions can be associated with ADHD?

There are a number of conditions that can co-occur with the diagnosis of ADHD. In fact, it is rare for a person to have only ADHD. Because of the likelihood that other problems may be present, it is recommended that these conditions be considered when developing a treatment plan. Frequent co-occurring conditions are described as follows:

- *Learning disabilities:* A high percentage of individuals with ADHD also have learning disabilities. A learning disability should be viewed as a separate diagnosis from the ADHD diagnosis. ADHD is not considered a learning disability, although a child may have both. Dr. Bruce Pennington (1991) supports the finding that a reading disability is a distinct disorder. His research has supported the theory that the syndromes of ADHD and reading disabilities are transmitted on separate genes. A learning disability could be in one or more areas. These include basic reading skills, reading comprehension, written expression, basic math skills, math reasoning, oral expression, and listening comprehension. For certification of a learning disability, most states require that a significant discrepancy be present between the person's intelligence and his or her academic achievement on an individually administered test (based on standard scores). However, it is suggested that an underlying processing disorder be documented also. For example, if a child has a learning disability in the basic reading skills, a phonological coding problem should be documented. In other words, the absence or presence of a discrepancy should not be the sole reason for diagnosing a learning disability.

- *Language and communication disorders:* It has been suggested that approximately 50% of those children who have been diagnosed with ADD demonstrate some type of language disorder (Love and Thompson, 1988). It has also been noted that ADD is the most frequent psychiatric disorder associated with deficits in speech and language (Baker and Cantwell, 1977). Given these findings, it is usually recommended that a language evaluation be completed when determining whether a child meets the diagnostic criteria for ADHD, particularly the inattentive type.

- *Emotional problems:* It is not uncommon for individuals with ADHD who have never been diagnosed and have gone untreated to be more likely to have emotional problems. Russell Barkley (1995) noted that up to 45% of children diagnosed with ADHD have at least one other psychiatric disorder, and these children may display more symptoms of depression, low self-esteem, and anxiety than other children.

- *Tourette's syndrome:* Tourette's syndrome is a genetic disorder manifested primarily by the presence of motor and vocal tics. The involuntary expression of swear words (coprolalia) does not have to be present in individuals with Tourette's syndrome. David E. Comings, director of the Department of Medical Genetics at the City of Hope Medical Center, reported that 60 to 80% of patients with Tourette's syndrome have ADHD. He and his colleagues believe that Tourette's syndrome is ADHD with tics (Comings, 1996).

- *Disruptive behavior disorders:* Many children who are diagnosed with ADHD will progress to more severe behavioral disorders, such as Oppositional Defiant Disorder (ODD) or Conduct Disorder (CD). It is hoped that with appropriate treatment these more severe behavioral disorders may not surface. While most children with ADHD will be oppositional at times, a diagnosis of ODD is more severe and the individual demonstrates a significant amount of defiant or oppositional behaviors. These include excessive arguments with authority figures, defying adults' requests or rules, appearing overly angry and losing his or her temper easily and often, and being vindictive. An individual with a CD diagnosis will demonstrate more extreme antisocial behaviors. These include behaviors that occur at a higher rate than would be expected of individuals of that age, such as deliberately destroying others' property, stealing, lying, being physically cruel to animals, running away from home, or skipping school regularly. A psychiatrist or mental health professional knowledgeable in the management and treatment of these behavioral disorders should be consulted if these conditions are present.

? *What treatments are effective for children and adolescents with ADHD?*

Although there is no cure for ADHD, there are a number of interventions that have been shown to be helpful to the family and the child or adolescent with ADHD. Research suggests that the most effective treatment involves a combination of medication and behavioral treatments at home and at school. William Pelham and his colleagues have demonstrated that this combined treatment approach offers more benefits than either treatment alone (Pelham, 1989). Possible treatment components include the following:

- *Medication:* This topic will be discussed later in this chapter.

- *Behavior management at home and at school:* This book will specifically address home situations in Chapters 2 through 7 and Chapters 9 and 10. School management will be presented in Chapter 8.

- *Parent training:* Studies support the efficacy of parent training programs in decreasing noncompliant behavior in children as well as improving the confidence level of parents (Pisterman, et al., 1992).

- *Environmental management:* Suggestions for the classroom environment will be presented in Chapter 8 and for the home environment in Chapters 3 and 4. There I suggest proactive classroom and home conditions that have been demonstrated to reduce the likelihood that behavior problems will occur in these settings.

- *Academic remediation or instruction:* If children or youth have specific learning problems in addition to ADHD, these deficits must be addressed. Specific suggestions, as well as what is required by law, will be presented in Chapter 8.

- *Social skills training:* An estimated 50 to 60% of children with ADHD have been shown to experience some form of social rejection from their peer group (Guevremont, DuPaul, and Barkley, 1990). Social skills training groups are frequently used with the child with ADHD, and better results appear to occur when the focus of training is on each child's specific problems. In addition, unless there are strategies built into the training that allow for a great deal of practice and feedback, it is unlikely that the child will generalize what has been learned in the group setting to the natural setting.

- *Home–school collaboration:* After years of working with school personnel and parents, I have concluded that children demonstrate improved behavior and academic skills when there is good communication and collaboration between the two settings. Chapter 8 will present information on the issues involved in this collaboration.

- *Cognitive–behavioral therapy:* Steven Hinshaw, at the University of California at Los Angeles and at Berkeley, has investigated the integration of behavioral and cognitive–behavioral interventions for the last 15 years (Hinshaw, 1996). As a part of a total treatment program, techniques that include self-monitoring strategies and anger management training show promise. Adolescents and adults with ADHD have used "coaches" to assist them in setting goals, getting organized, monitoring their productivity, and evaluating their behavior and performance. There are several nationally recognized coaching training sites. The Ch.A.D.D. organization (954-587-3700 or http://www.chadd.org) can provide information on these training sites.

- *Individual psychotherapy:* Not all children or adolescents who are diagnosed with ADHD will need individual psychotherapy provided in the traditional approach (i.e., where children or adolescents assume the primary responsibility for their progress). However, therapeutic intervention that is provided by a mental health professional who approaches treatment from a broad systems approach has been found to be beneficial to many children, adolescents, and adults with ADHD (Robin & Foster, 1989). In this approach, the mental health professional serves as the case manager for the family and communicates as needed with those who may have a role in the problems to be targeted for improvement. In this treatment, the case manager first helps the individual with ADHD and the family identify the problems (e.g., homework completion, school behavior, academic performance, peer relationships, anger control, family relationships). Next, the therapist guides the family in determining the problems that are priorities for intervention. As a plan is developed, the person who should assume responsibility for each part of the intervention is determined. For example, if homework completion is the problem being targeted for improvement, the family will determine the *child or adolescent's role* in the treatment (e.g., neatly writing assignment in book, completing assignment at home, returning completed assignment to school), the *parents' role* in treatment (e.g., purchasing another set of books to remain at home, providing the prearranged reward when assignments are completed and returned to school), and the *teacher's role* (e.g., teacher checks that assignments are written correctly in the assignment book, checks all assignments each day, informs the parent when assignments are missed). This approach tends to be more effective when the mental health professional understands ADHD and feels comfortable developing treatment from a behavioral perspective. In many situations, treatment consists of 10 to 15 sessions, with a gradual reduction in the frequency of the visits after the initial 10 to 15 sessions have been completed. These follow-up sessions usually occur once each month, then once each quarter, then twice per year if the family is doing well. As in other forms of intervention, it is advisable to reduce gradually the dependence on this person rather than abruptly stopping the treatment.

The model of intervention designed should reflect the child's own pattern of strengths and weaknesses, as well as the severity of his or her problems. For example, some individuals may need interventions to address behavior problems, but others may need interventions to address social functioning, self-control, or academic deficits. The plan of treatment should be individualized and provide youths and their families with the necessary tools to address their needs. Many parents have found that they need someone who can assist the family and the child in identifying the appropriate interventions. Often an objective case manager can help the family make decisions related to treatment. The case manager could be a pediatrician, a special education teacher or tutor, a psychotherapist, or another professional. This individual needs to have a thorough understanding of ADHD and its impact on the child's functioning. Although it is unlikely that all the treatment can be provided by this professional, this person should be able to view the situation globally and assist the family in finding appropriate services or interventions.

? *Will my child need medication?*

Medication, as a part of treatment, can be highly effective. It has been found, however, that medication dosages can be reduced and sometimes eliminated when other interventions are used to treat the symptoms of the disorder. While stimulants are most widely used for treating children with ADHD, there are other medications that are less frequently used. Approximately 80 to 90% of children with ADHD receive stimulant treatment at some time during their childhood (Bosco & Robin, 1980). It has also been demonstrated that more than 90% of children with ADHD will likely have a positive response to Ritalin or Dexedrine (Elia, Borcherding, Rapoport, & Kayser, 1991). It should not, however, be the sole form of treatment, and it should not be viewed as a way of controlling the child. In some cases, improvement with medication has allowed the child to remain in the regular classroom rather than go to special education for instruction in small groups. However, it should be noted that medication will not make up for lost skills in the academic areas. If skills are missing, remediation should occur. If medication is properly administered and managed, there is evidence to suggest that improvement may occur in all or some of the following areas:

- Improved classroom academic productivity and accuracy (Carlson, Pelham, Milich, & Dixon, 1992)

- Improved ability to solve problems (Douglas, Barr, Amin, O'Neill, & Britton, 1988)

- Decreased aggressive behavior (Hinshaw, Henker, Whalen, Erhardt, & Dunnington, 1989)

- Enhanced anger control (Hinshaw, Buhrmester, & Heller, 1989)

PSYCHOSTIMULANTS

It has been recognized for some time that stimulant medication can have short-term positive effects for children who are diagnosed with ADHD. The stimulant that is tried first will depend on a variety of factors (e.g., age of individual, other conditions in addition to the ADHD, the severity and type of symptoms). Of the four stimulants, methylphenidate (Ritalin) is the most frequently prescribed. It has been investigated through carefully controlled studies for over 30 years, and it is considered to be the stimulant with the fewest side effects.

Methylphenidate

RITALIN: Regular Ritalin takes about 30 minutes to take effect, and it lasts about three to four hours. Most individuals need two or three doses per day. Some parents report that the generic form differs in its effect; however, this has not been thoroughly investigated. Possible side effects include loss of appetite, stomachaches, headaches, weight loss, and tics. Side effects stop once the medication is stopped.

RITALIN SR (slow release, long acting): Ritalin SR comes only in a 20 mg tablet. It usually takes effect within 60 to 90 minutes and lasts about six to eight hours. The same side effects are possible as for regular Ritalin. Some families have reported that the medication does not appear to release evenly. In addition, some individuals report an improved response when a small dose of the short-acting Ritalin is given with the one SR tablet in the morning. This appears to help "jump-start" the effects.

Dextroamphetamine

DEXEDRINE: It usually takes effect in 30 minutes and lasts about three to four hours. Possible side effects include loss of appetite, sleep problems, irritability, headaches, stomachaches, and tics. Most individuals need two to three doses per day.

DEXEDRINE SPANSULES: It usually takes effect in 60 minutes and lasts approximately 6 to 10 hours. Because of the length of time needed to take effect, some individuals have taken a small dose of the short-acting form with the long-acting form the first thing each morning. The same side effects as in the short-acting dose have been reported. A number of health professionals are finding that Dexedrine Spansules work well for the adolescent because medication may not be needed during the day while at school. It may not, however, remain effective long enough for the adolescent to complete homework assignments; thus, a second dose is sometimes used.

Pemoline

CYLERT: This medication may take two weeks to take full effect, and the tablets last from 12 to 24 hours once it takes effect. Usually only one dose is given each day. Potential side effects include headaches, stomachaches, and sleep problems. Because rare instances of abnormal liver functions have been reported with this medication, blood tests are recommended prior to taking the first dose to check the liver functions and then once every six months while taking the medication. Many physicians find this medication useful for adolescents because they do not need to take medication while at school.

D/L-Amphetamine

ADDERALL: This is a newly approved psychostimulant. It is usually given if Ritalin or Dexedrine is not effective and is typically given twice a day.

ANTIDEPRESSANTS

In some cases, individuals may be unable to tolerate stimulants, do not have a positive response to stimulants, or have other conditions (e.g., depression, anxiety, compulsive behaviors) that would warrant treatment in addition to stimulants or to replace the stimulants. In these situations, tricyclic antidepressants (TCAs) may be useful. Unlike stimulants, antidepressants can provoke individuals to build up a tolerance, and the medication may need to be stopped for a while and begun again a few months later. The most frequently prescribed antidepressants used in the treatment of ADHD are described below.

Imipramine

TOFRANIL: Most physicians begin with one dose (1 to 5 mg/kg of body weight) before bedtime, increased as needed and recommended by the physician. This medication must be taken daily and should be stopped only under the supervision and direction of a physician. It usually takes about two weeks to take effect and lasts 12 to 24 hours. Common side effects include dry mouth, constipation, dizziness, fatigue, and stomachaches. Most physicians recommend a baseline electrocardiogram (EKG) before taking the medication the first time.

Desipramine

NORPRAMIN: This is typically begun with one dose (approximately 1 to 5 mg/kg of body weight) in the morning and increased as needed and recommended by the physician. This medication should be taken daily and must be stopped gradually while under the supervision of the physician. It usually takes three to five days to take effect and lasts about 12 to 24 hours. A baseline electrocardiogram (EKG) is recommended prior to taking the first dose. Commonly reported side effects include dry mouth, blurry vision, fatigue, and stomachaches.

Amitripyline

ELAVIL: The same procedure of dosing is followed with Elavil as with Norpramin and Tofranil. It must be taken daily and stopped slowly and only under the direction of the physician. Reported side effects are similar to those with the other antidepressants.

Fluoxetine

PROZAC: There are fewer studies and less is known about the use of this drug in treating the symptoms of ADHD in children. It has been primarily used in the treatment of depression in adults. In addition to using it with children who have mood disorders (depression, anxiety), it has also been reported to help reduce aggression and impulsivity in children with ADHD (Barkley, 1995). This medication, as with the other antidepressants, is typically prescribed and monitored by a psychiatrist.

ANOTHER MEDICATION

Catapres

CLONIDINE: This drug is used primarily as an antihypertensive medication for adults with high blood pressure. It comes in a tablet and patch form. While it is being used to treat children with serious aggression and impulsivity, it has not been shown to improve attention in the child with ADHD (Hunt, Capper, & O'Connell, 1990). Evidence has suggested caution in its widespread use with children with ADHD. The prescribing physician must carefully and closely monitor Clonidine.

? *How do you know if your child will need medication?*

The fact that your child has a diagnosis of ADHD does not mean that he or she should automatically be prescribed medication. In particular, it is typically not recommended for children younger than four years of age. For parents of younger children, parent training in child management strategies is strongly recommended. In addition, some physicians, as well as many parents, want to try other psychosocial treatments before medication is tried. These treatments could include many of those listed in this chapter.

If after having a thorough physical examination, you and your child's physician decide to try medication, it needs to be closely monitored to determine the appropriate dosage. The dose of medication is conditional on a number of factors that you and your physician will discuss. If your child is prescribed either methylphenidate or dextroamphetimine, your physician may also allow you the flexibility of having "drug holidays." For example, if your child is fine at home on the weekends and is not required to complete tasks or activities that require sustained attention and/or interactive group participation, medication may not be needed at home. Common practice by most physicians is to prescribe the lowest dose possible and to give it only when needed to obtain the desired results. However, parents should not adjust the dose prescribed by the physician without the physician's advice.

Final Comments

As you can determine after reading this chapter, ADHD is a complex condition, and each child may present with different impairments and subsequently need different treatments. ADHD is a condition the child was born with, and it was not caused by something the parent did or did not do. Since there is no one test that can be used to make the diagnosis, a team of professionals should be involved in the assessment process. The type of treatment recommended will depend on the severity of the condition and the number of other conditions present in the individual. For example, Matthew's treatment consisted of a multimodality treatment plan that included medication, social skills training, parent training in child management issues, environmental changes in the school setting, a behavior plan at school, academic remediation for his weaknesses in reading, and a consistent plan for home–school communication. Because his impairments were multifaceted, his family also used a mental health professional to help them coordinate and prioritize the treatment. Not all children with ADHD will need this intensive of a treatment plan, but by identifying a professional who can coordinate the services needed for your child, you may reduce or eliminate problems.

Where Do I Begin?

If I could say just one thing to parents, it would be simply that a
child needs someone who believes in him no matter what he does.

—Alice Keliher

A parent of an adolescent recently shared with me the story of her son who is now 16 years of age. John had participated in our Summer Treatment Program as a 12-year-old. He was sharing with his mom how difficult it was for him to get motivated to complete his school assignments. He said he thought he just wanted to drop out of school and get his GED. His mother was quite accustomed to his impulsive comments and began to express the reasons he should remain in school. John responded, "Oh, Mom, I just need some incentives to do my work! Getting a grade six weeks from now isn't enough. I need something now." As I spoke with John's mother, I shared with her that John had actually acquired a very good understanding of himself and what he needed in order to succeed. In spite of the fact that he had gained some maturity in the last four years, he recognized that he continued to need, at times, a reward that would help to motivate him to reach a goal.

? Is there any hope for me in learning to parent my child?

This book will introduce you to parenting approaches that will help you better manage your child's behavior. While the principles presented are effective with all children, parents of children with attention-deficit/hyperactivity disorder (ADHD) or other disruptive behavior disorders need to implement the principles presented in this manual with greater consistency. It is very difficult to parent a child with ADHD, and many parents feel that they are failures as parents when their child's behavior is inappropriate. All too often, their feelings of self-worth are based on how well their children behave. While you did not cause your child's ADHD, you and your child can acquire skills that will help to improve your child's behavior. With increased knowledge of the strategies presented in this book and opportunities to practice these strategies with your spouse or a friend, you will be able to help your child display more appropriate behavior.

In order to see real changes in your child's behavior, it is critical that you and your spouse, "significant other," child's grandparents, or others who might help in the parenting role agree on important parenting issues. If you disagree, do not air this disagreement in front of your child. If it is something that cannot be discussed later in privacy with your spouse, ask your spouse to go with you to a private area of the house (e.g., bedroom, on the patio) to discuss the issues in question. Use humor in doing this, and avoid approaching your spouse with a superior, "know-it-all" attitude.

? Why does my child act like this?

Common questions parents frequently ask themselves are "Why does my child act like this?" "My other children aren't this much trouble." "He's driving me crazy!" "Why me?" "What have I done wrong?" "Does he act this way because his dad and I are divorced?" While these questions are important to the parent, it is helpful for parents to understand that children come into the world with certain temperaments. Chess and Thomas (1987) hypothesize that "differences in temperament in the newborn and the very young infant are biologically determined, but then the infant's temperament is influenced by her interaction with her parents, which may either intensify or modify her original temperament" (p. 25). While you have little control over the type of temperament your infants will have when they are born, you can control other environmental factors in their lives. Some babies, from birth or even before birth, are very active and fussy, and may experience problems in their eating, sleeping, quality of mood, and attention as infants. Other babies have few problems and are easy to raise, sometimes appearing to raise themselves.

Chess and Thomas (1987) reported from their earlier studies that there were three patterns of temperament and that most children fit into one of these patterns. They reported that about 10% of the children from their sample had a *difficult temperament*, 40% had an *easy temperament*, and 15% had what is described as a *slow-to-warm-up temperament*. Other children showed other combinations of attributes that did not fit into a neat label. Chess and Thomas (1987, p. 32) characterize "easy" children as demonstrating regularity of their functions (e.g., eating, sleeping, eliminating), a positive approach to most new situations, easy adaptability to change, and a mild to moderate intensity of mood. "Difficult" children were characterized on the opposite end of the spectrum; they experience irregularity in biological functions, negative interactions when in new situations or with new people, difficulty adapting to change, and intense moods that may be frequently negative. "Slow-to-warm-up" children demonstrate a tendency to respond negatively to new situations and people and adapt slowly. Usually these children have a lesser tendency toward irregular sleep and feeding schedules. When upset, these children tend to withdraw rather then explode or have temper tantrums.

It has been further documented that approximately 70% of the babies with difficult temperament experience behavior problems in childhood and adolescence, and only 15 to 18% of the babies with easy temperament have behavior problems in childhood and adolescence (Jenson, 1995). We all know that it is not easy to parent the difficult-temperament child. As Jenson noted in his research, children with disruptive behavior disorders (those with difficult temperaments) comply about 40% of the time with a parent's request. If you have a child with a difficult temperament, it will take significant effort and consistency to help your child maintain a higher compliance rate and reach adolescence without major problems. This book will present principles that will result in a higher compliance rate and, hopefully, permit you to enjoy your parenting experiences regardless of your child's temperament.

? If my child is predisposed to a certain temperament, is there anything I can do to improve our interactions?

The information provided on temperament is not meant to imply that all children who are diagnosed with ADHD have difficult temperaments. Many children who later obtain a diagnosis of ADHD were reported by their parents to have an easy temperament. Many of these parents have reported that everything was going well until their child began crawling or walking. At that point, they had to lock all the doors, place the trash container on top of the kitchen cabinets, and keep an eye on their child 24 hours a day. There has been evidence, however, in support of a high correlation between difficult-temperament babies and a diagnosis of Oppositional Defiant Disorder (ODD).

When followed, the principles and activities presented in this book will increase the likelihood that positive behaviors will occur more often in your child. You will be introduced to different approaches that work when your child argues, is noncompliant, throws a temper tantrum, or demonstrates other inappropriate behaviors. There is no magic formula to "cure" your child. The goal is for you to learn approaches that will help you to manage your child's behavior from day to day and from year to year in order that your child can mature into a successfully functioning adult.

This book will not provide you with all the answers you will ever need to raise your child, but the principles and suggestions presented will be a good resource for you now and in the years ahead. Because of the severity and nature of the problems your child presents, you may also need family or individual counseling to address other problems. Although the information presented in this book is based on sound principles that have been investigated through research and lived through experience, it should not replace the insight you gain from a psychotherapist. The skills upon which this book is based are the principles of *social learning* that Gerald Patterson and his colleagues began over 30 years ago (Patterson, 1975). Many of you are aware of these principles, but it will be helpful to review these. These principles will be used and developed further throughout this book.

? *What are the principles of social learning, and why are they important for me to know?*

PRINCIPLE 1

Before punishment can be effective in changing your child's inappropriate behavior, you must first build in many opportunities for your child to receive your focused attention as well as your positive feedback. Most parents immediately want to know how they can stop a behavior they think is "bad," rather than follow this important principle. Commonly asked questions include "How can I stop my child from arguing?" "My child never listens to me. How can I get him to listen to me and to do what I say?" "How can I get her to complete her chores at home?" "I have to tell him the same thing over and over. Why can't he do it the first time I tell him?"

First, answer the following question: Are you giving your child enough of your focused attention and positive feedback in order that changes in her or his behavior can occur? Ask your spouse to keep track of the number of positive statements you make in one evening. When you are not aware of the evening your spouse selects, your spouse should count the number of positive comments or actions you give to your child. At the end of the evening your spouse can share this with you. If you are not giving sufficient positive feedback, and the only time you are interacting with your child is when your child misbehaves, the approaches discussed in the punishment chapter will be much less effective.

Before identifying approaches to address problem areas, stop now and list three behaviors you want your child to do more often or to start doing. Remember that these are not behaviors you want your child to stop, such as "Stop picking at your sister," "Stop arguing with everything I say," or "Stop waking up in such a bad mood." Think instead of "start" behaviors. These behaviors should be phrased positively. Examples of "start" behaviors are "I want my child to do what I say the first time I say it," "I want my child to say something positive each morning when he gets out of bed," or "I want my child to put his dishes away after he has finished eating." List in the space below three behaviors you want your child to start or to do more often.

1. _____

2. _____

3. _____

If you believe that most of your interactions with your child are to correct her or his inappropriate behaviors, begin the habit of "special time" with your child. This is a structured approach to giving your child focused attention. It is a practice most families find very enjoyable. This time should be given daily and be one-on-one. Your child does not have to earn this time. This is your child's time simply because she or he is your child, not because she or he had a good day at school. The following procedures were adapted from a program begun at Michigan State University, Department of Psychology–Psychology Research.

Special Time

1. Select a time each day that is to become your "special time." Set aside at least 10 minutes for this activity. This works best if it is the same time each day (e.g., immediately before bedtime, while dinner is cooking, before school in the morning). The time of the day is not as important as the consistency of maintaining the same schedule. "Special time" should be a priority, and it should be interrupted only in the event of an emergency. If your child is older than 9 years, you do not have to choose a structured time each day, but find time each day to do something your child enjoys or join in an activity in which she or he is engaged.

2. Talk to your child in advance and explain the program. Tell your child that she or he can select what to do or play during the "special time." As a parent, you will do whatever is suggested unless it is harmful to your child or to someone else, destructive, or against your house rules.

3. Do not allow other children or adults to be involved in this child's "special time." Other children in the family can have their own "special time." This time is "special" because the two of you are together. This approach to giving your child focused attention for 10 minutes often helps to reduce the amount of time during the remainder of the day that the child demands your attention. It also provides an opportunity to develop a ritual or routine within your house that will help build self-esteem and special memories.

4. On the day you begin the "special time," casually approach your child and ask if she or he has decided on the activity for the "special time." If your child has difficulty deciding, you might select an activity the first day. Do not pressure your child to decide or criticize the selection made. You may decide to talk or read a book the first day. After your child becomes more comfortable with this time, she or he will likely provide you with many ideas.

5. When your child begins talking, use active listening techniques. Do not give lectures or talk too much. Remember that it is your child's time to talk about what she or he chooses. Avoid asking too many questions or giving commands.

6. If your child uses this time to ask for special privileges, first listen to the request. Do not get into an argument over these requests. Just listen to the reason that she or he wants a special privilege, offer your reasons, and then tell your child you will think about it and discuss it tomorrow during your next "special time."

7. Occasionally during "special time" give your child specific, positive feedback: "I am really enjoying our conversation." "You have some really great ideas." "You are a really great reader. You read with such expression. I'm really proud of your progress in reading."

8. If your child begins to misbehave during this time, first try turning away and looking at something else (active ignoring). If the misbehavior continues, tell your child that "special time" is over and leave the room. Offer an opportunity to return to "special time" if the misbehavior stops. If the behavior becomes aggressive or too disruptive, you will need to implement a consequence.

PRINCIPLE 2

When a behavior is followed by a reward (reinforcer), the behavior is more likely to occur again. Does this work for adults also? If you have cooked a great dinner and your spouse compliments your efforts, as well as the product, you will be more likely to cook your spouse a meal again. The more immediate the reward, the greater its effectiveness. When you want to see a behavior occur more often, initially reinforce it every time it occurs, and then gradually reduce the number of times you reinforce it to keep the behavior continuing. If the appropriate behavior stops occurring, it may be that you stopped the praise too quickly, and you may need to increase the frequency of the praise for the time being. There are several types of reinforcers.

Social Reinforcers. These rewards do not cost anything. We all need these, regardless of our ages. These rewards include activities such as a hug, smile, verbal praise, pat on the back, high-five, or thumbs up. The more specific this praise, the more effective it will be.

It is more effective to comment to your child, "You did a great job putting away your toys!" as opposed to, "You were good today." This helps your child know the specific behavior you like; thus, the child is more likely to demonstrate this behavior again. If you just tell your child that she or he had a "good day," your child may not know specifically what made it a "good day." Your definition of a "good day" may be different from your child's definition of a "good day"; thus, you are not specifically reinforcing the behavior of "putting away the toys." If you want your child to put away the toys again, immediately and specifically reinforce the behavior.

For each of the "start" behaviors you listed earlier in this chapter, begin today to give your child praise each time it is observed. Below are suggestions on the techniques that are effective in giving praise.

- *When your child demonstrates one of the "start" behaviors you have listed, immediately give praise and attention.* For example, when your child is playing appropriately with his sister, tell him, "Michael, I really like the way you and Amy are sharing your toys."

- *When giving verbal praise, describe what you like about the behavior rather than make a general statement.* For example, "Eric, you did a great job of putting on your clothes all by yourself."

- *Avoid the desire to give a backhanded compliment.* While Eric was putting on his clothes by himself for the first time, you noticed that his shirt was on backward. Do *not* say, "Eric, good job. You put your clothes on by yourself, but you put your shirt on backward." If you want him to try again tomorrow, avoid these little comments at the end of the praise. You can work on the other at a later time.

- *Praise small steps toward a larger goal.* The large goal might be that Eric will be able to put on his clothes correctly without assistance or without being told to do so. In order to reach this large goal, reinforce the small steps along the way, rather than only praising when the ultimate goal is reached.

- *Be sincere when giving praise.* If you have a low rate of praise (as counted by your spouse), praise may not feel natural at first. The more frequently you give praise, the more comfortable you will become. Praise should not be false flattery but sincere praise. Your child will be able to discern the difference.

- *Vary your praise statements.* If you use the same praise comment each time the behavior occurs, your child will eventually tune you out. For example, a friend of mine consistently uses the word "super" to his children as well as his friends. After numerous "super" comments, we have all tuned him out.

- *Fit the praise to the child's age and to the things he or she likes.* Male children who are older often do not like the "gooey-mushy" praise, especially if it is given in the presence of other boys.

Activity and Material Reinforcers. Typical activity or material rewards include playing basketball with Dad, inviting a friend to spend the night, choosing the dessert for dinner, and checking a book out of the library. It is important to continue to give the social reinforcer (e.g., praise, hug, pat on the back) when you give a material or activity reward. Often, activity rewards are great for children with a high activity level, and you are encouraged to identify as many of these as possible when giving your child rewards.

An appropriate use of this type of reinforcer could be as follows: Immediately upon arriving home from school, Emily began her homework. After she worked quietly in her room for one hour, her dad suggested to her, "Emily, let's play a short game of basketball. You have been working so hard on your homework that I think you deserve a break."

Stop now and develop a list of activity and material rewards. Watch and listen to your child during the next week. Try to identify incentives that your child likes. Make a list of 10 to 15 rewards. These can be activity or material rewards. Suggestions are listed in Table 2.1. Identify activities that your child enjoys rather than always using material rewards. Keys to selecting appropriate rewards for this list include the following:

- The size of the reward should fit the child and the behavior. For example, it would be inappropriate to list "a trip to Disney World" for cleaning the bedroom one time. The items listed should be ones that will be easy to provide and that do not cost a great deal of money.

- The reward should be something that your child finds reinforcing. If your child hates basketball, do not list "play basketball with Dad." While this may be an activity you want your child to enjoy, if she or he does not currently like it, it will not be a good reward. To identify rewards your child likes, observe and listen to her or him. What does she or he select to do when there is free time? What does she or he select to buy when at the store?

- The rewards listed should not be activities or materials that are available at other times during the day. For example, if you allow your child to control the remote on the television all the time, this would not be a good reward. If, on the other hand, your child is rarely given this privilege, and you know she or he enjoys it, this would be an excellent reward.

- The reward should be something that can be given close to the time that the appropriate behavior has occurred. If the child, especially a young child or a

TABLE 2.1
Positive Reinforcers That Cost Little or No Money

Jump on the trampoline with Mom or Dad
Stay up 1/2 hour later
Catch fireflies with Mom or Dad
Have a friend spend the night
Spend the night with a friend
Sleep downstairs or in the tent in the yard
Lie on the trampoline with Mom or Dad and look at the stars
Have control of the remote for one hour
Get a 15-minute backrub by Mom or Dad
Do one less chore for each day for a week
Select a movie to rent
Eat dinner in the family room
Play a game with Mom or Dad
Sit at the head of the table for a day
Make a trip to the pet store
Play basketball with Mom or Dad
Select the dessert for dinner
Have an indoor picnic with a friend
Go bike riding with Dad or Mom
Select the cereal for the week
Drink hot chocolate with Mom before bedtime
Take the camera to school and take pictures of my friends
Select the radio station to listen to while in the car
Push the cart in the grocery store
Have breakfast in bed
Mom or Dad makes my bed for two days
Plan the menu for the day
Bake cookies with Mom or Dad for the class
Read in bed for 30 minutes

child with ADHD, has to wait one week for a reward, you are less likely to achieve the desired results.

- Surprise your child occasionally with a reward. For no reason at all, occasionally, just give your child a positive reward. All good things that happen to your child do not have to be earned or planned in advance. Your child needs some positive experiences just because she or he is your child.

Token or Point Reinforcers. Tokens or points can be exchanged for material or activity rewards. A social reinforcer should be paired with the tokens or points also. Earning tokens or points by themselves is not enough. The tokens or points must be cashed in for something in much the same way as you cash your check.

In working with one mother on a behavior management system for her child, the mother informed me that she used the "point system," but it wasn't working. The child was continuing to exhibit inappropriate behaviors at a high rate. I asked this mother what her child did with the points after they were earned. She stated, "Nothing. She just earns points." With most children who are ADHD, just earning points will not work to change behavior. To be effective, the points must be "cashed in" for something more rewarding. The reward needs to be motivating to the child to change behavior. As John suggested at the beginning of this chapter, the grades did not sufficiently motivate him to turn in his work. He needed a more powerful motivator. You will learn this approach to improving behavior in Chapter 6 of this book.

PRINCIPLE 3

Behavior changes slowly. Just because you are giving positive feedback when your child demonstrates an appropriate behavior, and even if you have implemented a reward and consequence plan, behavior still changes slowly. The building of positive habits to replace old negative habits does not occur overnight. It requires that you remain consistent in your reinforcement and parenting plan. This will be discussed further in Chapters 5 and 6.

PRINCIPLE 4

To weaken some problem behaviors, actively ignore them (Clark, 1989). You should *not* ignore some behaviors (e.g., destruction of property, aggression), but you can develop a procedure for planned ignoring of certain behaviors. The following guidelines may help you create your own plan.

First, determine whether your child is demonstrating this behavior simply to get your attention. Common behaviors that are included in the attention-seeking category are whining, begging, pouting, breath holding, mild temper tantrums, and crying with the intent to punish you. You should not use active ignoring for behaviors that can cause harm to you or to others. Use active ignoring only for those behaviors that are clearly aimed at getting your attention (Clark, 1989).

Second, if you decide that you will ignore a specific behavior, you must ignore it each time the behavior occurs. Talk about this decision with other members of your family. If they will join you in ignoring this behavior, the change will tend to occur more rapidly. To ignore a specific behavior requires a great deal of willpower and determination on your part. If you do not believe that you can consistently ignore this behavior, active ignoring will not be successful in stopping this behavior. If you give in to your child's desires after she or he has cried for 10 minutes, your child has trained you to do what she or he wants. In this situation, you are rewarding the inappropriate behavior, and the inappropriate behavior will be more likely to occur again.

While shopping in the grocery story last week, I observed a mother interacting with her five-year-old. He was screaming because his mother would not buy him the desired candy bar. After five minutes of embarrassment, she gave in and said, "Oh, here. Stop your screaming!" The child, in this situation, learned that screaming in a public place will get you what you want. The mother reinforced the screaming; thus, it will likely occur the next time that they go to the store.

Third, to actively ignore, you will demonstrate a behavior, such as turning your back to your child, reading the newspaper, or leaving the room. By doing this behavior, you will be informing your child that you will not reward his or her behavior.

Next, at times, when you decide to ignore the inappropriate behavior, it may get worse before it gets better. Don't give up. Check the first three guidelines to ensure that you are using the correct procedure. Have your spouse evaluate your active ignoring procedure. If all the guidelines are followed, continue the plan. Eventually, your child will learn that the whining does not achieve the desired reward (e.g., your attention, a candy bar), and the inappropriate behavior will stop.

Finally, when your child stops the inappropriate behavior and demonstrates an appropriate behavior, immediately reinforce the positive behavior. For example, Allison is whining in the grocery store because you will not allow her to buy her favorite cereal. After several minutes of whining and your continued ignoring, she talks to you in a normal voice. Immediately, give her focused attention (e.g., talk to her). This does not mean that you should give in to her desire for her favorite cereal, but that you should provide her with attention when she ceases to whine.

PRINCIPLE 5

To stop some inappropriate behaviors, you will need to punish them when they occur. We have found in working with children who display a high rate of disruptive behaviors that positive reinforcement alone will not stop all negative behaviors. A plan for appropriate punishments or consequences will be needed also. You will need a balanced plan of action: positive reinforcement for appropriate behavior and consequences for inappropriate behavior. Appropriate forms of punishment will be presented in Chapter 5.

PRINCIPLE 6

Reward the behavior that you want to replace the inappropriate behavior. For example, Brandon usually grabs toys from his sister, but this time he shares his toys with her. Praise him immediately when he shares his toys. "Brandon, what a nice job of sharing. How do you feel when you share?" Sometimes, in an attempt to praise the child's behavior, the parent inadvertently does the opposite. For example, an incorrect approach to praising the replacement behavior would be: "It's about time you started sharing." This will not result in improved behavior over time.

PRINCIPLE 7

Provide your child with many opportunities to practice new behaviors. This will give your child the time and the opportunity to form new and positive habits. It may be helpful for you and your child to role-play certain problem situations. For example, if your son frequently turns the television channel while his sister is watching a show, have him practice the appropriate way to change a channel. Try the following steps:

1. Model the appropriate way to ask for a channel change.

2. Have your child practice the appropriate way to ask to change the channel. In this step, the practice should be supervised by you with specific feedback.

3. Praise him each time he handles the situation appropriately.

Occasionally, opportunities for repetitive practice are helpful. I recall the time my father scolded me for slamming the back door when running into the house. After numerous reminders, he decided it was time for me to practice the replacement behavior for slamming the door. He informed me that I was to go to the back door and close it appropriately 100 times. As I recall, the next time I ran into the house, I remembered the appropriate way to close the door because I had formed a new positive habit.

PRINCIPLE 8

Anticipate problem behaviors. Most of us *react* to a situation or a problem rather than *proactively* think of approaches to avert a problem. As in basketball, the successful team has both a good offense and a good defense. One alone is not sufficient to win a national championship. The defense is the *reactive* approach to a situation, and the offense is the *proactive* procedure used to prevent problems from occurring. Often, problem behaviors can be avoided if the parent plans ahead. For example, if you know Rob is tired and hungry after school, don't take him shopping with you on this trip. Another proactive approach would be to review the rules of "riding in the car" immediately before your trip. Or plan something for your child to do while he must ride eight hours in the back seat with his sister. By anticipating problem situations and developing a proactive plan of offense, you can avert many problems. Plan ahead!

Final Notes

Attempting to teach children new behaviors takes time, but it also requires that parents be good role models for their children. The old saying, "Your actions speak so loudly, I can't hear what you're saying," applies here. If you model yelling and screaming when you don't get your way, it is likely that your child will do the same. However, it should be noted that even if you are a "perfect parent," your child may still exhibit problem behaviors that need changing. Remember that 70% of the difficult temperament babies grow up to have behavior problems in childhood and adolescence if appropriate treatment is not implemented. The reverse of this is that 30% will not have severe behavior problems. The specifics to apply these principles will be developed as each chapter unfolds. Be a good model for your child this next week. Follow these tips from Kersey (1987). Try to be

- *big* enough to say you're sorry when you jump to conclusions or blame someone else when the fault is yours;
- *brave* enough to say "no" when it would be easier to say "yes"—especially when you know that your "no" will make you unpopular and your child angry;
- *courageous* enough to take a good look in the mirror and honestly evaluate the self you see;
- *strong* enough to put forth the effort to become the person of your dreams;
- *self-disciplined* enough to work hard for the goals that you think are important;
- *secure* enough to look for and affirm the good you see in other people;
- *patient* enough to let your child learn from his own mistakes;
- *loving* enough to let him suffer the consequences of his actions;
- *honest* enough to tell the truth when your child comes to you with a question;
- *sensitive* enough to "be there" when he needs you;
- *relaxed* enough to realize the importance of spending time alone with your child each day;
- *intelligent* enough to realize that he has much to teach you if you will only listen;
- *calm* enough to stop in the midst of deadlines and rush hours to watch the sunrise, listen to the ocean, smell the spring rain, and feel the softness of sand beneath your feet;
- *accepting* enough to realize that your child is a separate person—with needs, qualities, strengths, and weaknesses unlike yours and unique to him;
- *capable* enough to cope with daily obstacles—to attempt to solve problems and not just complain about them;
- *thoughtful* enough to show respect to your own parents and other older people by sacrificing your time and energies for them;
- *smart* enough to rest when your body is weary, exercise when it is stiff, eat when it is hungry, and stop when it is full;
- *kind* enough to be concerned about the needs of others; and
- *wise* enough to remember that if you want your child to grow up to possess these noble traits, it will be necessary for him to see them first in you (Kersey, 1987, pp. 224–225).

Techniques for Improving Compliance in Your Child

The best and most beautiful things in the world cannot
be seen, nor touched . . . but are felt in the heart.

—Helen Keller

Chapter 2 emphasized the importance of giving your child focused attention and positive reinforcement. If you are consistently applying these principles in your parenting, there is a greater likelihood that your child will demonstrate more appropriate behavior. As you may recall, the positive reinforcement you give your child must occur more often than the negative feedback you give. As is the case with many of us, we find it easier to identify negative behaviors in our children than positive ones. You may also find it easier to name the behaviors you want your child to stop doing, rather than the behaviors you want your child to do more often or to start doing.

? *Why is it so important to give my child positive attention, when I don't have to do this for my other children?*

You may ask, "But how can I stop Michael's bad behaviors?" You, like most parents, want to know what forms of punishment are needed to stop these inappropriate behaviors. Appropriate forms of punishment or consequences are necessary to change some behaviors, and these will be presented in Chapter 5. For now, however, it is critical that you form the habits of providing your child with ample positive feedback and giving your child focused attention when appropriate behavior is being demonstrated. If your child only gets your attention when she or he does something wrong, you will likely see an increase in these inappropriate behaviors. Why?

> ▶ In a recent home visit, the counselor returned with a videotape of her time with the family. Mark, a 5-year-old, was running through the house chasing the dog while his mother was cooking dinner. In an attempt to get him to stop, she yelled to him from the kitchen each time he ran by the kitchen, "Mark, stop running!" He stopped running for a while, but then he began again with the addition of teasing the dog. His mother scolded Mark, "Mark, leave the dog alone! He's going to bite you." This stopped for a few minutes, and then Mark ran out the back door chasing the dog, pulling his blanket full of toys. She stopped her cooking, ran to Mark, grabbed him by the arm, and sat him in the time-out chair. Within 10 minutes Mom was frustrated and angry. Mark was upset and in tears.

What was happening in this situation? First, each time a negative behavior occurred, Mother gave Mark attention. Even though it was negative attention, it was still attention. Second, she failed to give him attention and/or praise when he complied with her request to stop a behavior. In this situation, Mark was being rewarded with Mom's attention each time he exhibited an inappropriate behavior. Thus, these behaviors continued. Other factors that may have contributed to Mark's high noncompliance rate were the high frequency of commands and the high rate of "stop" commands. These factors and their relationship to noncompliance will be described later in this chapter.

? How can I find the time and energy to focus on my child's positive behaviors?

Because our lives are usually so busy and full of hassles and conflicts, it becomes much easier to focus on the negatives rather than the positives in a child's behavior. Similar to the expression "Catch 'em being good," the idea of *celebrating the positives* (McLaughlin, 1995) involves focusing on your child's appropriate behavior, on the interesting and worthwhile personality qualities, and on the accomplishments in various areas of your child's life. This approach also involves celebrating the positive relationships that your child enjoys within your family and with others outside the family. To aid you in this process of celebrating the positives, follow the suggestions of Dr. Joseph McLaughlin (1995), a child clinical psychologist:

- You and your spouse (or another adult if someone else is involved in parenting your child) identify the qualities in your child that you perceive as being positive.

   List your child's special talents. _____
   _____

   How does your child make himself or herself or others happy? _____
   _____

   What is easy to love about your child? _____
   _____

- Next, identify, recognize, and celebrate accomplishments in your child's life. These may appear to be small, but each child has at least a few in each area listed below.

   What has your child accomplished at school (at camp) today or this week (e.g., made a new friend, finished homework, swam without water wings)?
   _____

   What has your child done to make family life more satisfying today (e.g., put clothes in the dirty clothes hamper, said thank you for the snack, hugged you before going to school)? _____
   _____

- Identify ways to celebrate relations in your family. One way that was suggested in Chapter 2 is the daily "special time." If you have not tried this approach to building your parent–child relations, review this section and try it for one week. *Beginning* a routine, such as a daily special time with your child, is the hardest part of developing a new habit. Once you make the commitment to *begin* this habit, continuing it may be easier. Acknowledge episodes of positive interaction between siblings. When these are observed, celebrate these relations by giving praise or by sharing in their enjoyment. What are some recent memorable instances that are examples of good relations (e.g., your two children playing ball together, coloring you a picture)? If you are unable to identify these instances, create activities that will facilitate this exchange. You may take the family on a bowling outing or a picnic, complete a puzzle together, or take a family walk in the park. For special memories to occur, they do not need to be expensive vacations or long excursions. In fact, most of our children with ADHD tend to enjoy the experiences that are brief because they are better able to maintain a high level of interest and appropriate behavior. When the activity loses its novelty, your child may be more likely to exhibit inappropriate behaviors.

• Identify times when your child has demonstrated positive relations with friends. Recognize these and celebrate these times with your child.

With whom does your child get along? _____

_____

Are there settings in which your child feels comfortable with her or his peers—school, church, scouts, sports events, participation in hobbies? Encourage your child in these areas and provide her or him with opportunities to continue these activities. Avoid using the threat of "grounding" a child from participating in activities in which she or he derives a positive sense of self-worth. For example, if your child is particularly talented in basketball and has recently made the school's team, avoid using this privilege withdrawal as punishment for poor grades.

Do you provide your child with opportunities to enjoy the friends she or he has made? If you are worried that these may result in inappropriate behavior, begin this new experience with more direct supervision from you and then gradually reduce the amount of supervision as your child is able to handle it. Avoid placing your child in a "no win" situation. Set up the peer interaction for success, especially the first time this is attempted. List activities that you may plan during the next month that will permit your child to be with her or his friends.

_____

_____

❓ *Okay, I'm doing this positive thing, and my child still doesn't mind me. What now?*

▶ My child never seems to listen to me. When I talk to him, I always seem to be screaming or scolding him for not completing a task that I have just given him. I've tried to find something positive to say to him, but I can't get beyond the screaming. What do I do?

Does this sound familiar? Sometimes it's helpful to stand back from the encounter with your child and really listen to what is happening. Some families have found it helpful to leave a cassette recorder on for an hour or two in the evening to listen to the communication that is occurring. To identify potential problems in your family's communication, listen for phrases commonly used in your home. Or ask your children to join you in keeping a running list of the words and phrases spoken frequently during the next week. Do these phrases focus on activities that foster positive communication, or do they focus on activities that limit real communication, such as the ones that are commonly used when watching television ("What's on?" "Turn the channel." "It's my time to watch . . .")? Phrases that are more likely to enhance communication within your home are more open-ended statements, such as "How was your game?" "What was the most exciting thing that happened?" "Did anything exciting or different happen at school (camp) today?"

Parents of children with more disruptive behaviors should be able to give clear commands and instructions to their children. Often, the way in which a command or a request is given to a child will determine whether the child complies.

▶ During one of our Summer Treatment Programs, I had one 7-year-old boy named Alex who was extremely oppositional. When a staff person told him to do something, 90% of the time he did not follow through with the command, even when given the command the second time. His counselors were extremely frustrated with Alex's high rate of noncompliance.

In an attempt to determine approaches that might help, I met with his parents. His parents were asked if they had the same problems at home. They responded, "No, he always does what we say." In shock, I asked them to please share with me their secret in order that we could implement it in our treatment program. His father responded, "Oh, he does what I say after I've told him about 10 times and then I yell at him in my mean voice."

What was happening in this situation? Alex had learned that his father did not mean what he said until he yelled at him on the 10th time. He was not required to comply with his parents' command the first time or even the second time it was given. Alex had about a 10% compliance rate with his parents as well. It was no wonder we were unsuccessful in our attempts to improve his compliance rate.

❓ Are there strategies for improving my child's compliance rate?

Before providing you with information on the techniques needed to improve your child's compliance, let's first determine when a command should be given. A command is given when you want your child to stop a behavior immediately and you believe that a simple request will not achieve the desired result. Many times, your child may not comply with your command because you are giving bad commands. William Jenson (1995) and his colleagues have found that children with ADHD or other disruptive behaviors have about a 40% compliance rate. In our Summer Treatment Program, "noncompliance" is one of the problems parents most frequently mention. If you implement the suggestions in this book, your compliance rate should increase. Types of commands that frequently have a low compliance rate because they are bad commands are as follows:

1. *Vague command:* A command is vague when you do not specify an observable behavior. For example, "Stop that bad attitude, Michael!" A specific observable behavior was not noted in the command. Michael's definition of a "bad attitude" may be different from your definition. What specific behaviors are included in the "bad attitude"?

2. *Question command:* Questions are okay as long as you can accept "no" for an answer and when the question is not intended to be a command to stop something. For example, the following is not a command: "Clay, would you clear the table?" Clay has the option of responding, "No, I'm coloring right now." If he does not have the option of saying "no," don't ask the question.

3. *Extended command:* An extended command is one in which the parent makes statements that provide a rationale for reasons that a command should be followed. By the time the parent has completed the rationale, the child has forgotten the command (and sometimes the parent has forgotten also). For example, "Clay, pick up your toys

from the living room. We are going to have guests in a few minutes, and I don't want them to see all this mess on the floor. Someone might fall and get hurt. You're always leaving things lying around."

4. *Chain command:* Stringing a series of commands together that the child cannot follow or remember will typically result in noncompliance. For example, "Clay, go brush your teeth, pick up your toys from the living room floor, call your sister for her special time with her dad, put on your pajamas, and get your book for our 'special time.'" Most children with ADHD cannot follow these commands that are chained together. Clay may be able to remember one or at the most two of these commands.

5. *Let's command:* Including in the command a "let's" phrase is a bad command. A *let's* phrase is one in which the child infers that you are going to help her or him when this is not what you intend. For example, "Let's put your bike away." Your child may still be waiting in the driveway for you so you can help to put the bike in the garage. Did you intend to help?

6. *Repeated command:* A command given 5 to 10 times, as Alex's father had in the first example, is a poor command. For example, "Come to the dinner table! I said come to the dinner table. You are really making me angry, come to the dinner table! This is the last time I'm going to tell you!! If you don't come now, I'll throw your food out to the dog!!!"

7. *Harsh command:* This command is given in a harsh, sarcastic tone of voice. It usually results in anger rather than compliance. This command usually occurs when the parent has had a particularly difficult day.

You and your spouse should listen to the types of command you frequently give your child. Are you giving any of the bad commands listed above? If so, you can change and, in the process, increase your child's compliance rate. The following are suggested guidelines for giving appropriate commands:

1. *First, get your child's attention.* Don't yell the command from the kitchen while the child is watching television. Move close to your child, say her or his name, and request that your child look at you. Most teachers and parents give commands from too far away. The most effective commands should be given within 3 feet of the child (Kehle, Clark, & Jenson, 1996). Mark's mother in the first story failed to get his attention prior to giving the command; thus, a high rate of noncompliance occurred.

2. *Give one command at a time.* Give a direct, simple, and clear command—for example, "Put your shoes on your feet before going outside."

3. *Follow the command with 3 to 5 seconds of silence* (Kehle et al., 1996). Much of the time, commands are interrupted within the 5 seconds. To be effective, give the command, and wait 5 seconds (in silence). The command should be the last thing your child hears: "Your grandmother will be here in five minutes. Holley, place your toys in the toy box." Wait 5 seconds in silence.

4. *If your child has not followed the command within these 5 seconds of silence, give your child an "I need you . . ." statement* (Reavis, Jenson, Kukic, & Morgan, 1993). This procedure is used in our work with children who are more defiant. These children tend to respond better to an "I need you . . ." statement than to a "You better do it now, and I mean it" type of statement. Most of the children who are more oppositional will respond negatively to the latter statement. With many children who exhibit disruptive behaviors, it is often best to avoid the "If . . . then" warning: "Holley, if you do not pick up your toys, then you will have to go to time-out." Many times these warnings will result in an escalation of disruptive behavior. An "I need you to place your toys in the toy box" appears to work better. The child is not backed into a corner. When Holley complies with this request, her parent should immediately praise her. If she does not comply with the command, her parent would implement the pre-arranged consequence.

NOTES

Many parents report that their child must always have the last word when they give a command. One approach to reduce the likelihood that the "last word" will be negative is to teach the child an acceptable response and then provide the child with time to practice it. For example, Jason, a 10-year-old, and his mother agreed to the following response as being acceptable:

MOTHER: Jason, please empty the trash before dinner.

JASON: I've got you covered. (He proceeded to complete the chore.)

It should be noted that compliance rates decrease when the number of commands is too high. Thus, it is important to avoid giving commands unless they are absolutely needed. How many commands do you give in one day to your child? Observers have found that mothers of children without behavior problems give 17 requests per hour, whereas mothers of children with behavior problems give 27 per hour (Forgatch & Patterson, 1989). Count the number of commands you average in 1 hour on a given day. Then, calculate your child's compliance average by counting the number of times she or he complies the first time a command is given. (A reproducible Compliance Monitoring Chart is in Appendix C.)

▶ During the second week in one summer's program, we had one 10-year-old boy who maintained a low rate of compliance (23%). After observing the counselors interact with him, it was determined that he was being given too many commands. Brian was told to "Sit up straight," "Stop picking your nose," "Look at the counselors," or "Stop playing with the rocks." Before a plan was implemented, the counselors were instructed to count the number of commands given by them in each hour of the day, and then to count the number of times he complied with the command the first time it was given. On average, Brian was given 32 commands per hour. The number of commands he was given was too high; this was likely one of the reasons for his low compliance rate.

The first assignment was to reduce the number of commands that were given to Brian. Through a series of steps (e.g., giving him immediate positive feedback when he demonstrated appropriate behavior, giving more "start" commands rather than "stop" commands, setting up a contract between the staff and Brian), his counselors were able to reduce the number of commands he was given. After six weeks of intervention and by implementing strategies to reduce the number of commands he was given, his compliance rate had increased to 72%.

? *Often when I give my child a "good" command and tell him to stop doing something, he just argues with me. What do I do?*

Another method that will improve compliance, as well as increase the positives in your home, is to provide your child with more *start* requests than *stop* requests/commands. A start command involves redirecting the child from the negative behavior to a positive, opposite behavior. For example, a start command for a child who is running through the house while her sister is studying would be "Go to your room and start your homework," or "Justine, walk in the hall quietly." Study the following list of stop commands and notice the replacement start command:

Stop Commands	**Start Commands**
"Stop flipping the television channels."	"Place the remote on the coffee table."

"Stop jumping on the bed."	"Go outside and shoot some baskets."
"Stop talking during the movie."	"Listen really carefully and tell me how many times the man says the word *what*."
"Stop asking when we will get there."	"Please look at the map. We are here (pointing to the map). How long do you think it will take us to get to here (point to the destination)?"
"Stop teasing your sister."	"Scott, I need you to set the table for dinner."
"Stop putting your feet on the table."	"Put your feet on the floor."

When told to "stop" a behavior, children tend to become argumentative. When you give your children "start" commands, you will tend to have fewer arguments and will get them involved in something positive. It serves no purpose to engage children in arguments. Just give them a task that will stop the inappropriate behavior. At times, it is extremely difficult to pause for a few minutes to think of a "start" command. If your child is running into the street, you can't wait too long to inform the child to "Stop, don't run into the street." But many times, problems can be avoided if you form the habit of giving more "start" requests. For example, last summer I overheard a counselor say to a child, "Stop humming that song!" What do you think the child did? He started humming another song. If she had given a start command, she may have been more successful. "Scott, I need you to read the next paragraph," or "Scott, I need you to hold the whistle for me."

If your child is extremely noncompliant, you may benefit from spending some time with your child practicing compliance. By using this method, you can train your child to develop the habit of compliance. To train your child to comply with your requests, do the following:

When your child is playing appropriately alone, sit with your child and give several simple requests. "Give me a red crayon," "Pass me a magazine," "I need a fork; please get me one." After each request, allow your child time to respond and then specifically praise her or him for following your request. "Thank you for giving me the magazine." In the beginning, try several of these training sessions. Make sure the requests are simple and that your child is in a positive mood. Don't do this training immediately after the two of you have had a fight. And most importantly, remember to provide *specific* praise after your child complies.

If you have implemented the approaches suggested in Chapters 2 and 3, you should be observing some changes in your child's level of happiness, as well as in her or his compliance rate. In the next chapter, you will be presented with several other approaches that will continue to improve the interactions within your family.

A Suggestion for Parents

William Jenson (1995) suggests that parents should occasionally surprise their children by rewarding them for compliance. He suggests that when you randomly reward your children for compliance, their compliance rate will likely increase. For example, periodically give your children a command, such as calling them into the house when they are playing outside. When your children come to you, give them a treat and tell them to go back outside and play. If you do this occasionally, you will see that the compliance will be higher when you really need your children to come into the house to complete a chore for you.

An analogy for those of us who fish is the occasional reward we receive when fishing. If you truly enjoy fishing, you know that you will not catch a fish each time you go fishing. This occasional reward does not stop you from fishing. The reality that you receive an occasional reward actually increases the likelihood that you will go fishing again. Remember, however, that an occasional reward should *not* be used when you are implementing the structured behavior change program or point system described in Chapter 6. If it states in the program that a reward is given each time a certain behavior occurs, this reward must be given as indicated.

Final Notes

Continue to identify ways to celebrate the positives in your child. All of our children have special talents and ways to make us happy. Make a conscious effort to identify these, encourage them, and celebrate them within the family. Don't get so caught up in the daily hassles of parenting and working that you lose sight of the fun and enjoyment your child can bring to the family.

Carefully listen to the communication between you and your child. Do you give too many commands? If so, identify ways to reduce the number you give. The number may be reduced by (a) giving your child "good" commands; (b) giving more "start" requests than "stop" requests; (c) using an "I need you . . ." statement when your child does not comply the first time a request is given; (d) praising your child immediately when she or he complies with a request; and (f) following with a prearranged consequence when the command is not followed the second time.

Other Methods To Increase Good Behavior

> There comes that mysterious meeting in life when someone acknowledges who
> we are and what we can be, igniting the circuits of our highest potential.
>
> —Rusty Berkus

Chapter 3 discussed celebrating the positives in your child and giving appropriate commands. If you are using these techniques, you may have discovered that your child is more likely to do what you say. While your child is not perfect, there should be improvement if you are consistently using these techniques in your parenting. Even if your child has an easy temperament, it is still unlikely that he or she will comply 100% of the time. Did you comply with your parents' requests 100% of the time? A 100% compliance rate is an unrealistic expectation; thus, if you have this as a goal, you need to challenge the legitimacy of this goal for your child. Changes in behavior are slow to emerge because the former behaviors have developed into habits over many years. A 60% compliance rate may be acceptable for a child with ADHD or for one who exhibits other disruptive behaviors. The average child with ADHD has a compliance rate of about 40%, while the "goody-goody" child has a compliance rate of approximately 80% (Jenson, 1995).

One father in one of our parenting groups recently shared with the group the following experience. He had tried unsuccessfully to get his 8-year-old son to wear his sneakers rather than his sandals to camp. He had tried reasoning with him and explaining the importance of wearing shoes (e.g., You can play ball better when you wear your sneakers." "You might hurt your toe if you wear your sandals."). He had given up and said the battle just wasn't worth the effort. The morning after the session on the topic "Commands," the father decided to give his son a "good command" to get his son to do what he wanted him to do. He told his son politely, "David, we need to leave for camp in five minutes. Please put on your sneakers." David gave the usual excuses and said that he would just wear his sandals. Dad responded, "I need you to put on your sneakers." To Dad's surprise David immediately put on his sneakers. David gave no comment, just immediate compliance.

Not all the experiences of parenting will be this easy, and not all the techniques presented in this book will work this quickly. However, you are likely to have a higher compliance rate only if you issue commands when they are absolutely needed and when they are appropriate.

❓ *Our biggest problem is getting my child ready for school each morning without a battle. How can we improve this time of the day?*

As suggested earlier, you need a good offense as well as a good defense to experience balance in your parenting. Always reacting (defensive game plan) to situations will not substantially decrease conflict in your home. Include strategies that will improve your offensive game. An effective offensive strategy that is useful in decreasing conflict between parent and child is the establishment of routines. Establishing a routine requires a commitment by you to teach the routine to your family and to value it sufficiently until it becomes well established and useful for your child and your family. This commitment requires time and effort. The time and effort needed in the establishment of a routine can be thought of as an investment in your family's well-being. If the investment is made wisely, it will return dividends of decreased family conflict and an increased sense of competence for your child (McLaughlin, 1995). To develop a routine, first determine situations or times that are particularly problematic for you and your family. Problem times for many families include getting up in the morning, going to bed, and completing chores. Once you have determined the problem to attack, establish a step-by-step routine that could be followed by all members of the family. By involving your child in the planning process, a more positive approach to establishing routines will likely occur. The more your child is involved in this decision-making process, the greater likelihood that she or he will be invested in it working. A few common situations for which routines are appropriate are listed below (McLaughlin, 1995).

GETTING READY

- Set a regular time to get up. To involve your child or to get her or him invested in the routine, take a special trip to the store so that your child can buy an alarm clock.

- Assign regular responsibilities for your child and other members of the family (e.g., make the bed, brush teeth, put breakfast dishes in the dishwasher). When assigning these responsibilities, determine what is developmentally appropriate for your children to do. Don't do for your children what they are capable of doing for themselves.

- Include in the routine self-help responsibilities that will maximize your children's skills and that are within their ability level. For example, 6-year-olds can be responsible for putting on their own clothes, even though they may not put them on perfectly.

- After the job responsibility or routine has been successfully completed, acknowledge it and specifically praise the behavior. One effective alternative way to reinforce behavior is to talk about your child positively to another adult. For example, you might call the grandmother and tell her how well your child is doing. Remember to do this in a way that allows your child to overhear the conversation.

BEDTIME

- Set a regular time for bedtime. On weekends, you may decide to allow your child to remain up longer.

- Establish calming activities and habits. For example, after your child puts on pajamas, you could view a favorite video together for 30 minutes.

- Schedule a time for quiet appreciation of your child. This may be a good opportunity to schedule your "special time."

- The structure and consistency of a routine supports a sense of comfort and security for your child.

HOMEWORK

Additional techniques for homework completion will be discussed in Chapter 8.

- Decide on a regular place to complete homework.

- Let your child assist you in organizing the materials. You may visit the store together to select materials that will be needed for most assignments (e.g., pencils, crayons, markers, scissors). You may allow your child to decorate the container over the weekend prior to this routine beginning on Monday.

- Set a regular time to complete homework. If your child is involved in extracurricular activities, you may need some flexibility in this; however, keep to the routine if at all possible.

- Periodically check for progress in a positive way.

CHORES

- Assign consistent duties. Consider the age and ability level of your child before assigning chores. Often, we rob our children of many opportunities to build self-esteem because we think they are too young to complete certain chores. Let your children do what they are capable of doing.

- Shape the performance in the learning of chores. Implement the "I do, we do, you do" approach to learning new skills. In this approach, first the parent shows the child how to complete the chore (I do), next the child and parent complete the chore together while the parent is talking the child through the process (we do), and third, the child completes the chore without assistance (you do). I realized the importance of teaching chores through this approach when my son, who has ADHD, was in the army. He called home one evening and informed me that he had made the highest grade in his entire platoon on the parachute packing test. Since this was the first time Thomas had ever made the highest grade on any test, I asked how he had accomplished this. He responded, "Oh, it's just the way they teach here. The sergeant showed us what to do, then he told us what to do while we did it, and then I had to do it myself." As parents, we often spend too much time telling our children how to do something, when using the army way (I do, we do, you do approach) may work better.

- Provide your child with acknowledgment of her or his competencies. Be specific, such as "Mike, I'm so proud of you. You went straight to your room after dinner and started your homework. Way to go!" Remember that parents need to reward the effort as much as the actual product, especially for the child with ADHD.

- Appreciate your child's contributions. Be specific.

Select one area listed above and develop a written plan (or pictorial plan) for making it a routine. Remember that routines are more effective if the child is involved in creating the steps of the routine. When developing a routine, carefully consider your child's developmental and ability levels.

▶ One parent of a 7-year-old child with a serious language disorder, as well as ADHD, developed a routine with her son that used his strong visual skills and did not penalize him for his weak listening and reading skills. In developing Sam's morning routine, they talked about all the things he needed to do each morning to be ready for school by 7:30 A.M. His mother then took pictures of Sam completing each of the steps in his morning routine (e.g., getting out of bed, making his bed, eating his cereal, brushing his teeth, putting on his clothes, getting in the car). She then copied and enlarged these pictures at a local copy company. She sequenced these pictures with Velcro (with numbers below the picture) on her son's door. As he accomplished each step in the routine, he was permitted to pull the picture off the door and place it in his special basket. He was subsequently rewarded with 5 minutes of cartoon time for each step he had successfully completed. As the morning schedule became more routine, he no longer needed the visual reminders.

It is recognized that many of our children with ADHD struggle to complete the morning and evening activities. If your child is taking a short-acting stimulant, you do not have the assistance of medication to help your child through the completion of these routines. It is suggested that you first try the routine approach for the time of day that is problematic prior to speaking to your physician about medication changes. Some physicians have allowed the parent to awaken the child 30 minutes prior to the normal waking time to give the child medication. Thus, the child is better able to accomplish the morning routine. Disadvantages to using this approach are that (1) the time of the second dose at school will need to be 30 minutes earlier, and (2) the child may not eat breakfast because the medication may reduce the appetite. Thus, it is usually beneficial to try the routine plan prior to making changes in the medication. The routine plan may just work.

❓ Should we have house rules? Other families have them, but sometimes I think we have too many rules for our child with ADHD.

One approach to reduce the need for reminders for appropriate behavior and guidelines within the home is to establish *house rules*. House rules, if effectively established and working, will help reduce the overuse of commands. By the time children enter elementary school, they should be ready to follow appropriate house rules. House rules provide the child with a guide for appropriate behavior that is expected for each family member, parents included. It should be noted, however, that children must be reasonably compliant and cooperative before you can expect them to consistently follow house rules. If your children are not reasonably compliant, go back to the compliance training procedure suggested in Chapter 3.

When children approach the adolescent years, allow them to be more involved in the decision making for establishing house rules; however, there are some rules that are nonnegotiable. You and your spouse should determine the rules that are nonnegotiable prior to meeting with your preadolescent. Rules that are often nonnegotiable include issues related to drinking, using drugs, members of the opposite sex in the house without an adult, and aggression. Your family may have other rules that are nonnegotiable. There will be a number of areas that will be negotiable, and these can be discussed with your child. Below are the suggested steps for establishing house rules (adapted from Patterson & Forgatch, 1987, pp. 32–37):

1. Write down rules that your children already follow consistently (e.g., leaving phone messages next to the phone, making the bed before leaving the house each morning). When speaking with your children about house rules, you can compliment them on these areas. In addition, jot down several behaviors that require constant reminders.

2. At a calm and appropriate time, the entire family should meet to discuss the formulation of house rules. Inform your children that the family needs a few house rules

because you do not want to nag them about certain things and that you think this will make your home a happier place in which to live. Ask your children to think of several rules they think would make them and the family happier. Encourage them to state these as things they *want* rather than things they don't like—for example, "I want you to knock on my door before barging in," rather than "You always barge in my room when I'm writing in my private journal." Tell them you will be doing the same. Think of several behaviors that you must constantly remind your children to complete, and include these on a list. Make a *suggestion box,* ask the children to place suggestions in the box, and open it at the next family meeting (about 2 days later).

3. At the family meeting, spend a brief time discussing each suggestion. (Parents still have veto power because there are some rules that are nonnegotiable). Select 5 to 10 rules that are appropriate for the entire family. Select a couple of rules from the children also. House rules are rules that must be followed by everyone in the family, not just the children. If one rule is "Knock on a closed door before entering," then parents must follow this rule also.

4. Tape a list of the selected rules on the cabinet door, the bathroom door, the refrigerator, or another area in the home. Note: Preadolescents and adolescents may not like these to be posted in a highly visible area because they are embarrassed when their friends see them. You may choose to place them inside a cabinet door if you have adolescents at home.

5. During the first week in which house rules are used, family members should be observant of other family members and their adherence to the rules. In this stage, family members should only report a rule when a rule was not followed or when a rule was followed. During the first week, punishments should not be used; just be observers and make appropriate comments. For example, if one rule was "Put your dishes in the sink/dishwasher after each meal," and it was not followed, comment to the child or parent who did not follow the rule, "Dad forgot to put his dishes in the dishwasher, and Mom had to do it." Dad will then demonstrate the appropriate way to respond. "Oh, you're right, I got busy with my work and forgot. I'll do better next time." Encourage all family members to give positive feedback when they observe that a rule was followed. Through this approach, parents are modeling the appropriate way to handle constructive criticism without becoming defensive.

Work through the steps for house rules and develop these with your family. Good house rules should change as the needs of the family change. Possible reasons for change are that (1) everyone is following a rule consistently, and it is determined that a new rule should replace the old one; and (2) the children are older, and new rules are needed because of new situations. If your children are reasonably compliant, your home should have house rules. If they are not reasonably compliant, identify the breakdown and implement procedures to improve their compliance. Children should also understand that if a house rule is broken, a negative consequence should follow. A logical consequence tends to work best. After reading the next chapter, you can determine appropriate consequences for broken house rules. If there is no consequence, then the rule will likely not be followed—unless, of course, you have a child who complies with all the rules. Common house rules that have been developed by many of the families we work with include those shown in Figure 4.1. (A blank House Rule Form can be found in Appendix C.)

How do I get my child to express his feelings without yelling at me and everyone else in the family?

▶ When Rob arrived home from school, he started slinging his books and coat in front of his sister, Katie, who was watching television. He yelled, "I hate you, Katie. You always get your way!" His mother said, "That's no way to treat your sister!! Now go to your room and stay there until you cool off!"

House Rules

1. When someone is on the phone, refrain from interrupting the person unless it is an emergency. (With many of our children with ADHD, you will need to clearly define what you mean by an emergency.)

2. During the regular homework time, the house should be reasonably quiet, the television should be off, and only soft music may be played.

3. If a door is closed, knock and be recognized before entering.

4. Everyone must wear a shirt to the dinner table.

5. After the meal, rinse off your plate and place it in the dishwasher.

6. Before going to bed, all clothing articles, books, magazines, toys and games that are in the family areas of our home must be placed in the proper location. (This did not apply to the child's room for many families.)

We agree to abide by the rules established in our family meeting on _____.

Date

_____   _____
Parent's Signature   Parent's Signature

_____   _____
Child's Signature   Child's Signature

_____   _____
Other Signature   Other Signature

FIGURE 4.1. Sample house rules.

Did Rob's mother's response open the communication or close it? If you responded that it closed it, you are correct. Rob was not permitted to express his feelings at all, and this encounter with his mother taught him very little about an appropriate way to interact with someone when he is angry. He will likely become angrier because he assumes that his mom is not interested in his feelings. Occasionally, it may be necessary to give Rob a "cooling off" time before addressing his interaction with his sister. After allowing him a few minutes to "cool off," turn off the television and utilize the feedback technique to address his feelings:

MOM: Rob, I know you were really upset when you arrived home. Could you use your assertive (me) voice (if Rob has been in social skills training, he will understand this word) and share with Katie and me why you were so upset?

ROB: Katie is always watching television when I get home. I never get to watch my shows. Why does she always get to watch TV, and I always have to do my homework before I can watch TV?

MOM: That really bugs you that she gets to watch television, and she doesn't have homework in kindergarten, doesn't it?

ROB: She makes me so mad! I wish I didn't even have a sister; then I could always see my shows, and I wouldn't have to listen to her dumb shows.

MOM: You're angry with your sister because she gets to watch her favorite shows after school, and you don't feel that you get to watch yours. Is that right?

ROB: Yeah!

MOM: Can you and Katie help me find some solutions that would let you feel that you had some free time to do what you want to do and that the television would not interfere with your homework time? I think it will be a good idea if you both feel like you have some choice in what happens after school. Don't you?

By using this approach, Mom acknowledged Rob's feelings. She did not necessarily agree with his perceptions of what was happening, but he was permitted to express his feelings in a safe, accepting environment, where he knew that he was valued as a member of the family. If children are not allowed to openly express their feelings without fear of punishment, acting-out behavior or withdrawal may result. This does not mean that children should be allowed to verbally abuse a sibling or parent. However, it does take practice on the child's part and modeling on the parent's part for children to learn to express their feelings in a way that does not attack the other person.

The feedback technique described by Fitzhugh Dodson (1978, p. 61) is appropriate for parents to practice. Below are the steps Dr. Dodson recommends:

1. First, *listen carefully* to what your child is saying. Many of us do not carefully listen. We are too busy reading the newspaper or watching television. Your body language must indicate that you are listening. Look directly at your child and stop what you are doing if at all possible.

2. While you are listening, formulate in your mind what your think your child is trying to express.

3. Next, give feedback, using your own words, about the feelings your child was expressing.

At first, this technique may seem somewhat awkward or uncomfortable. With continued use, however, you will find it easier and more natural. Remember that *beginning* is the most difficult part when forming a new habit. And you will have to incorporate this into your daily encounters with your child in order for it to become a habit. In fact, your child may begin to utilize these techniques with others as a natural part of communication.

Practice the feedback technique described above with your spouse. First, listen carefully without comment, formulate in your mind what you want to say, and then provide your spouse with a paraphrase of her or his feelings. You do not have to agree with the feelings, and you do not have to use psychological terms ("I hear what you are saying"). You are just acknowledging your partner's feelings as being real, and you are using your own words. Don't you just hate it when you arrive home from work and the following exchange with your spouse occurs? You express the following to your spouse: "I'm really tired. I had a really hard day." In response to your statement, your spouse says, "I'm tired too." When this occurs, you may feel that you were not heard. The feelings you expressed were not acknowledged. It would have been more helpful if your spouse's response had been, "I'm sorry. What made it so difficult?" Then you would feel as if you were heard because your feelings were acknowledged. You did not need your spouse to solve the problem and go beat up your boss for making you work too hard; you just needed to be heard and understood. Sometimes, that is all our children need.

Listen and provide encouragement, and allow your child the opportunity to begin to solve some of her or his own problems. Children lose many opportunities to boost their feelings of self-worth when we solve all their problems or take care of all the negative situations. Your child may interpret your overinvolvement as informing your child that she or he is not capable of solving the problem, and you must do it.

All too often, parents tend to *react* to what the child said or did, rather than *respond* to what the child was trying to communicate. Dolores Curran (1983, p. 44) suggests four steps that can assist parents in learning to respond rather than react:

1. First, try to discover the reasons for the statement. Feelings may be hidden in the statement. Maybe Rob had failed a test at school, was in a fight with his best friend, or the teacher embarrassed him, and he is reacting to this rather than to his sister watching television. Discovering the reasons for the statement does not mean that you allow your child to verbally abuse his sister, but it may help you be more understanding of his bad mood.

2. Accept your child's statement as real. It was the way she or he perceived the situation; thus, your response will be to the perception of the situation, not necessarily what is reality. If you make a judgment at this point, communication could be cut off.

3. Be empathetic. Try to relate to the situation in a personal way. You do not need to top the situation by saying, "That's nothing; you should have seen how my sister treated me!" The key is to try to feel what the child is feeling.

4. If appropriate, help your child find a reason for the problem.

Each of us may need a reminder of appropriate listening techniques. We become so busy just dealing with the daily hassles of life that listening is often a lost art. Marion Forgatch and Gerald Patterson (1989, pp. 21–22) have recommended eight guidelines for improving listening skills. Practice these skills at home with your family. They can also be helpful when approaching a situation that may be adversarial or one that evokes a high level of stress. For example, before meeting with your child's teacher or attending a meeting relative to your child's performance in school, review these techniques and use them. A summary of these techniques is listed below:

1. When the other person is speaking, visualize what the person is saying in your mind. Give the other person time to talk. Don't interrupt, and don't speak until the other person has finished. This will help you to avoid responding impulsively.

2. Try to learn something from the speaker.

3. Stay focused on what the other person is telling you. Avoid thinking about what you want to say in response to the comments.

4. Ask questions that move the conversation along.

5. Try to match the other person's emotional state, unless it is hostile, and then do not match it. Remain calm.

6. Do not give advice unless you are asked.

7. Try to understand the other person's perspective.

8. Think before you respond. Your child may have problems with impulsively responding before thinking. Avoid this. Model appropriate behavior for your child. If you blurt out answers in the conversation, your child will be more likely to do this also.

Final Notes

Now that you have established proactive strategies, such as the use of routines and house rules, as well as some reactive strategies such as positive reinforcement, you are ready to implement other reactive strategies (e.g., punishment). You should continue practicing all the lessons presented thus far in order to have a balanced parenting plan.

Approaches for Stopping Negative Behavior

History has demonstrated that the most notable winners usually encountered heart-breaking obstacles before they triumphed. They won because they refused to become discouraged by their defeats.

—B. C. Forbes

Sometimes mistakes can be made in enforcing a mild form of punishment, and the results can be disastrous. The parents of a very bright 5-year-old boy with ADHD were ready to try time-out for the first time. The father placed Matt in time-out for hitting his sister. The time-out location was in the bathroom. After being in time-out for what seemed to Matt's father as a very brief time, he realized that Matt was very quiet. His father forgot about Matt because he was enjoying the peace and quiet while he was reading the newspaper. After some time, his father quickly walked into the bathroom after remembering his son was still in there. As he ran into the room, his father slipped on the bathroom floor and fell on his back. The reason for Matt's father's fall was that Matt had gotten bored while serving his time-out and had spread petroleum jelly over the entire floor.

? *I'm using mild punishments, and it doesn't seem to phase my child. The misbehavior continues. What's wrong?*

Many times, as in this situation, a mild form of punishment does not work because it is not enforced correctly. While many parents attribute the failure to the type of punishment selected or to their child's indifference toward punishment, the real reason may be due to the procedures used to implement the punishment. Effective punishment strategies that are useful for stopping or weakening negative behaviors will be presented is this chapter.

When used alone, punishments cannot increase good behavior. You must continue to be proactive in your parenting (e.g., establishing routines, setting house rules, giving "good" commands), and you must continue to react to the positives in your child by acknowledging and reinforcing appropriate behaviors. You should also avoid rewarding "bad behavior" (Clark, 1989, p. 21). For example, Joy and her daughter, Amy, were shopping at the grocery store. Amy began to whine and beg her mom for a candy bar. Amy continued to beg and cry more loudly. After 10 minutes of this behavior, the mother responded, "Oh, all right! You can have the candy bar. I'm tired of your crying." What happened? Mom rewarded the inappropriate behavior. Will this behavior occur again? Very likely, especially if Amy is rewarded with a candy bar occasionally. She does not have to get it every time for it to be a reward.

? Should I punish every negative behavior my child exhibits?

Some misbehaviors do not require the use of a punishment to get them to stop. Some behaviors are clearly aimed to get the attention of the adult. Many of these behaviors will be reduced or eliminated if the parent actively ignores the behavior. Active ignoring was presented in Chapter 2. Behaviors that may be clearly for the adults' attention include whining, begging, crying when not hurt, breath holding, and mild tantrums. Clark (1989) recommends the following guidelines for active ignoring to be effective:

- Briefly remove all attention from your child.

- Refuse to argue, scold, or talk.

- Turn your head and avoid eye contact.

- Don't show anger in your manner or gestures.

- Act absorbed in some other activity—or leave the room.

- Be sure your child's bad behavior doesn't get him or her a material reward.

- Give your child lots of attention when the bad behavior stops. (Clark, 1989, p. 23)

? When and how should I punish my child?

With some children, the parenting techniques suggested thus far may be sufficient to maintain a high rate of appropriate behavior. For other children, mild forms of punishment will be needed to stop some inappropriate behaviors. It has been clearly demonstrated that mild forms of punishment are more effective for the child with ADHD and for a child with other disruptive behaviors than harsh or severe forms of punishment. Mild forms will not emotionally damage a child, and most parents find that they can consistently enforce a mild punishment, whereas they are not as consistent with the more severe forms of punishment.

You must also remember that your child will imitate your behavior. For example, if you scream at your child or your spouse, it increases the likelihood that your child will exhibit this behavior also. If you tell a "white lie" to someone who calls you because you do not want to talk, it is likely that your child will imitate your behavior and lie in other situations. If you have a problem behavior, develop techniques to weaken it before your child mimics your behavior. Some parents may need professional help to make these changes, but it is critical that you change an inappropriate behavior in yourself before you can expect positive changes in your child for the same behavior. Children, as well as parents, can change inappropriate behaviors.

Before appropriate forms of punishment are presented, there are a number of critical factors to consider. Patterson and Forgatch (1987) present five guidelines for using punishment:

1. *It is better to use small punishments than big ones.* Many parents think that if they use severe punishments (long or harsh punishments) the behavior will change more quickly. This is not accurate. In this chapter, mild forms of punishment will be presented that can be used for smaller infractions that will, hopefully, prevent a larger problem or a crisis from occurring.

2. *It is better to use a small punishment each time the inappropriate behavior occurs.* Because many inappropriate behaviors have developed over a period of time, they

have become habits. In order to break these habits, you must use "many, small punishments, and many, small encouragements" for good habits to develop. Too often, we ignore the small inappropriate behaviors in hopes that they will disappear. As a consequence, they develop into larger problems, or the child is confused as to what is expected because one day you ignore the behavior and the next day you punish for the same behavior.

3. *Punishments should immediately follow the negative behavior.* The longer the time period between the misbehavior and the punishment, the less likely it is that your child will see the connection between the two, and the less likely she or he will be to change the behavior. Children with ADHD need this immediate response to a negative behavior more than your other children will need it.

4. *"Don't use threats unless you plan to back them up"* (Patterson & Forgatch, 1987, p. 171). Threats do not change inappropriate behavior, but the consistent use of punishment can. "NEVER threaten to use a punishment that you cannot, or will not, carry out" (p. 171). Examples of threats that cannot be carried out include: (a) "If you forget to take out the trash again, you will not be allowed to go outside for one week." (b) "You will be sent to time-out for the rest of the day if you don't stop that!" Are you really able to enforce these threats of punishment? If your child knows by your past actions that you will turn off the television when he and his sister fight over a show to watch, then you may say, "Stop fussing over the show to watch, or the television will be turned off." He knows this "threat" will be carried out because you have done this before; thus, the threat will likely result in changed behavior. These statements should be given in less than 10 seconds, with 10 words or less, with a 3- to 5-second pause after the statement. Do not say anything during this 5-second pause. If your child does not comply within this time period, you use an "I need you" statement: "I need you to find a solution to your dispute over the television show." If the child does not comply with your request, *immediately* turn off the television. If the child does comply within the time limit, *immediately* reinforce the appropriate behavior: "Thank you for working out a solution to your problem. You may continue to watch your show."

5. *"Limit your battlefields"* (Patterson & Forgatch, 1987, p. 172). Many parents make the mistake of trying to change all the child's inappropriate behaviors at the same time. This will not work. It is usually best to select one or two behaviors to change. Using routines and developing house rules may reduce the number of behaviors you must change. It may be wise to select one in which you and your child can see positive changes quickly. (This procedure will be discussed later in more detail.)

❓ *Okay, what types of punishment can I use with my child?*

As suggested earlier in this chapter, mild forms of punishment work better than severe, harsh ones. In one study, it was found that consistently using a 1-minute time-out for 3 weeks reduced problem behaviors by 61% in a group of institutionalized children (as quoted in Patterson & Forgatch, 1987, p. 168). Severe, long periods of isolation were not necessary to change these children's behavior. Several forms of mild punishment, when used consistently and appropriately, have been found to be effective for stopping or reducing inappropriate behaviors. These are discussed below.

VERBAL REPRIMANDS

The verbal reprimand is a statement indicating your disapproval of a specific act. As with commands, the number and frequency of reprimands will impact their success rate in stopping a negative behavior. When using verbal reprimands, the parent should express her or his feelings about the behavior and name the inappropriate behavior in as few words as possible. This reprimand is more effective if it immediately follows the misbehavior. The parent should use self-control and avoid using sarcasm or downgrading remarks.

▶ Dad discovered that his son, Brady, was using his tools without permission. He walked toward Brady, gave him eye contact, and stated, "Brady, I'm very disappointed that you got my tools without asking. Put them away in the tool box for the rest of the day. If you want to use them again, ask me first."

For some children, demonstrating disapproval through a verbal reprimand may be enough to change a behavior. This worked with my "easy temperament" child, Julie. Usually, a nod of disapproval or a soft reprimand was all that was needed to stop the inappropriate behavior. However, this did not work as well with Thomas. There are several signs that let you know that this form of mild punishment is not working. These signs may be that (1) the child only smiles at you when the reprimand is given and continues doing the inappropriate behavior; (2) the child talks back or argues with you; (3) the child has a temper tantrum; (4) the child mocks you; or (5) you find you are giving reprimands all day long, and the child continues to demonstrate the behavior. The more reprimands you give, the less effect they will have on changing behavior. This appears to be the case with families in which one parent stays at home with the child. Often, the parent who is with the child less will have a higher success rate in using reprimands.

There is no age limit for the use of this type of punishment; however, for many families with children who exhibit extreme oppositional behaviors, it may be only mildly effective in changing behaviors. When you know the reprimand is not working to change the behavior, you will need to use one of the other forms of punishment suggested in this chapter or some of the suggestions made in Chapter 6. Below is an example of an *inappropriate* verbal reprimand.

▶ Brady, you are a bad boy! Why do you *always* get into my things without asking? I'm sick and tired of you messing up my things. Your brother doesn't do this! What's wrong with you?!!!

The parent in this situation made several mistakes. First, he labeled Brady ("bad boy") and not the behavior. Second, he asked Brady a question, which could have given Brady the option to lie. When you know the child has done something that did not follow your rule, you don't need to ask questions. Just state the facts. Third, Dad compared him to his brother, which does not encourage positive relationships between siblings. Fourth, he did not specifically state the reason for the reprimand. He just said he was tired of his messing up his things or getting his things without asking permission. Lynn Clark (1989, p. 34) suggests that the parent should not allow this type of punishment to evolve into *nattering*. Clark defines *nattering* as a "combination of chattering, nagging, scolding, and complaining." To be effective, the reprimands should not be overused, and when given, they should be brief and specific and occur immediately after the misbehavior.

NATURAL CONSEQUENCES

A natural consequence is an event that naturally happens to your child following inappropriate behavior (Clark, 1989). Allowing a child to experience a natural consequence after an inappropriate behavior occurs is one effective way for your child to learn which behaviors are acceptable. However, a natural consequence should only be allowed when it will not result in injury to your child or to others or will not result in destruction of property. If your child is running into the street, you cannot use the natural consequence that may result in your child getting hit by a car. Of course, as parents, we want to protect our children from experiencing the natural hazards of life, but if we always do so, children will miss many opportunities to mature and learn from their mistakes. As Bob Brooks (1991, p. 93) states, "mistakes are experiences from which to learn rather than feel defeated by."

> ▶ When Phillip was in preschool, he hated wearing clothes. He preferred running around the house in his underwear. His parents decided to limit their battles; thus, while he was in the home, his mother and father made this rule, "When you come to the table to eat, you must wear your shirt and pants (shorts), or you will not be allowed to eat with the family." They thought that this would at least initiate some positive habit formation. This rule seemed to work for meal time, but they hadn't solved the problem at other times. Each morning before going to preschool, Phillip would find things to do other than get ready for school. A typical remark was, "Well, we're not eating, so I don't have to wear my clothes." His mother became very frustrated with him one morning, and she made a threat. "Phillip, if your clothes are not on by 8:15, we are walking out the door, and you will have to go like you are." Phillip's father, being a "good" psychiatrist, overheard the threat. He told Phillip's mother that she should expect Phillip to still be in his underwear by 8:15 and that she should follow through with her threat. As his father had predicted, Phillip refused to put on his clothes. At 8:15, Mother told Phillip to get in the car. Phillip grabbed a towel and wrapped it around his neck like a cape, and they proceeded to school with only a cape (towel) and underwear. They walked into the preschool classroom, the teacher looked at Phillip's mother and stated, "Is there something I need to know?" Afterward, Phillip was ready for school each morning because he had to suffer the natural consequence of other children laughing at him.

The natural consequence of going to school without clothing and being laughed at by other children helped Phillip to learn through a natural consequence. The battle to get dressed in the morning was over. Because many of us would never allow our children to experience such a lesson, our children may miss opportunities to learn from mistakes. Consider the following behaviors and a potential natural consequence for each:

Inappropriate Behavior	Natural Consequence
Emily refused to wear her coat to school.	The teacher would not allow her to play outside for recess because it was too cold.
Russ refused to wear shoes when he rode his bike.	He hurt his foot in the spoke.
Mary left her ball glove at home.	The coach did not allow her to play in the game.
Casey left his bike outside in the rain.	The bike rusted.
Tommy left his homework at home.	He obtained a "0" for that day or the teacher had him do it at recess.

LOGICAL CONSEQUENCES

When you cannot allow a natural consequence to occur, a logical consequence may be the next appropriate response. This type of consequence logically fits the misbehavior.

In other words, there should be a clear and reasonable relationship between the consequence and the inappropriate behavior. The consequence does not need to be severe to be effective. Examine the following logical consequences:

Inappropriate Behavior	Logical Consequence
Mikey left his bike in the driveway.	He was not allowed to ride his bike for one day.
Jody did not put his dishes in the dishwasher as the house rules required.	He had to wash the pots and pans for the evening's meal.
Sean put petroleum jelly on the bathroom floor while in time-out.	He had to clean the bathroom floor and buy another jar of petroleum jelly with his allowance.
Polly rode her bike outside the neighborhood without permission.	Her bike was put away for two days.
Jason intentionally broke a toy that belonged to his sister.	He had to give her his favorite toy or buy her a new one with his allowance.

Logical consequences can be effective for children as well as adolescents. As the child gets older, you must change the consequence to fit the child's likes and level of development. For a consequence to be effective, it must be something that the child values. For example, if your child does not like to ride her or his bike, depriving her or him of it would not be a good consequence. It should be noted, however, that many of our children would like their parents to think that they do not care. If you have selected to withdraw an activity or object that you know your child values, do not get into a power struggle or a debate over whether she or he cares or not. Just give the consequence immediately after the misbehavior occurs. If you cannot give it immediately, enforce the consequence as soon as possible.

BEHAVIOR PENALTIES

When you cannot think of a consequence that logically relates to the inappropriate behavior, a behavior penalty may be effective. Sometimes it is impossible to think of a logically related punishment. Behavior penalties should also be a mild consequence, and they are effective for any age, as long as the penalty has value to the child or adolescent. Grounding a child for one month is not an appropriate behavior penalty for "talking back." First, you are punishing yourself because you are grounded also. Second, it is unlikely that you can enforce this extended penalty. Third, short, brief punishments tend to be more effective than extended punishments in stopping an inappropriate behavior. Possible behavior penalties could include a fine, loss of privilege, or a brief work chore. When using a behavior penalty, state the specific misbehavior and the penalty to the child. Do not lecture; just briefly state these two facts.

▶ "Danny, your dad and I are concerned about the number of bad words (curse words) you have been saying. From now on, each time you or any member of the family says a curse word, that person must place a dime (quarter) in this jar. Do you know what I mean by a curse word?" Later, when Danny used a curse word, his father stated, "Danny, that's a curse word. Put one dime in the jar."

Clarifying with the child what is meant by a "curse word" is important. There may be a discrepancy between what the parent considers to be a curse word and what the child considers to be one. Remember that most children or adolescents with ADHD try to identify loopholes in what you say. Therefore, be clear in your definitions and use of behavior penalties. By clarifying these terms initially before implementing the penalty, you might avoid an argument. If a fine is used as a penalty, it should be based on the child's economic situation. For example, a parent may be required to pay a $1.00 fine, while a 5-year-old may only pay a nickel. If the child does not have money, give your child an opportunity to earn money by completing a job for you that is not one of her or his regular chores. Remember, if you want your child to stop saying curse words, the caregivers must also stop saying them. If you are using fines as a punishment, determine ahead of time what you plan to do with the money. It is not advisable to use it for an enjoyable activity for the family. One family gave the collected money to a charity.

Consider the following inappropriate behaviors and a potential behavior penalty for each:

Misbehavior	Behavior Penalty
Dolly lied to her parents.	She could not play with her Virtual Pet for 2 days.
Mancy said unkind words to her sister.	She was assigned a 5-minute work chore (e.g., clean toilet).
Sarah did not come home at the assigned time.	Sarah was not allowed to watch television for two days.
William made a sassy remark to his mother.	William was required to wash the dishes after dinner.

Five-minute *work chores* are an effective behavior penalty to use with the preadolescent or adolescent. Patterson and Forgatch (1987, pp. 189–196) describe the steps involved in using this behavior penalty:

1. Try to set the stage so you will not have to impose a work chore. For example, before making a request, create a friendly atmosphere.

2. Warn your child or adolescent only one time. If your child does not comply with your request after this one warning, a specific work chore will be assigned.

3. Don't lecture or argue.

4. Each time you are ready to make a request of your child, have in mind two work chores that you can immediately use if needed.

5. Impose no more than two work chores. If your child has not complied after two work chores have been given, withdraw a privilege.

6. The chore should be brief. It should take you no more than 5 minutes to complete; however, it may take your child longer. After the chore is finished, check it to see that it is done well, and avoid tacking on a "caboose" statement when checking the completion of a chore. For example, "You did a good job of cleaning the toilet; why don't you do that more often?" To provide a positive reinforcement, just state, "The toilet looks great! Thanks."

7. Stay out of the way while your child is completing the chore.

8. Stay calm and neutral. If you are having trouble remaining calm, develop your own self-control strategy to help you (i.e., counting to 20, taking several deep breaths, going outside for a few minutes, making a neutral phone call, such as to get the weather report).

Many parents are concerned that if work chores are given as a punishment, the child will not learn that she or he must also complete the other assigned chores. Work chores are different from chores that would be assigned because a child or adolescent is a member of the family. All of us should be responsible for certain chores in the home, and they should be matched to our ability level (e.g., a 5-year-old can place her or his dirty clothes in the clothes hamper). In addition, it is my opinion that the child or adolescent should not be paid to complete the regular chores. If you want to give your child the opportunity to earn money for the completion of work chores, these should be in addition to the regular chores that are required because she or he is a member of the family. It is important for a child to learn that we all have certain responsibilities because we live in a family.

Prior to using the assignment of a "work chore" as a behavior penalty, make a list of chores that take you only 5 minutes to complete. Do not include chores that are a regular part of the child's responsibilities within the home, and select chores that are within the child's ability level. Also remember that if your child finds these chores pleasurable, they are not effective as punishments. This is the reason that 5-minute work chores are more effective with the preadolescent or adolescent. Many young children enjoy completing chores for their parents. Chores that have been used with parents in our Summer Treatment Program include activities such as the following:

- Clean the toilet.
- Sweep the porch.
- Empty the dishwasher and put dishes in their proper location.
- Take the laundry from the dryer and fold it.
- Clean out the cat litter box.
- Vacuum the car.
- Pull weeds from the flower garden.
- Clean the window on the storm door.
- Clean the mirrors in the bathroom.

If you plan to use the assignment of work chores as one of your options for behavior penalties, stop now and take a trip through your house. List as many chores as possible that would take you 5 minutes to complete. Keep this list handy. Thus, when you must assign a chore, you will have several in mind.

TIME-OUT

The term *time-out* means time out from reinforcement. Time-out has been shown to be effective for stopping certain inappropriate behaviors in children who are between the ages of 2 and 11. Many of you are thinking, "Oh, I've tried time-out with my child. It doesn't work." Let me encourage you to read the instructions for using time-out and determine the possible reasons that time-out was not effective in weakening a past behavior. Try to remain open to using time-out as a mild form of punishment. It is far more effective in the long run than spanking. Time-out does work if it is appropriately used. If you follow the guidelines outlined below, and it still does not appear to work, read the questions in Table 5.1 for additional aids. The following guidelines will be helpful in successfully using time-out.

1. *Determine which behaviors warrant a time-out.* Both parents must agree on the behaviors that warrant a time-out. Behaviors that tend to deserve a time-out include those that are aggressive to another person (e.g., hitting people, kicking people, pulling hair), behaviors that are intended to result in the physical destruction of property (e.g., kicking door, knocking a hole in the wall, destroying toys, pulling down window blinds), and behaviors that occur because of a child's repeated refusal to comply with your com-

TABLE 5.1
Questions To Ask Yourself When Time-Out Is Not Working

1. Am I giving my child more than one warning before placing her in time-out?
   Most of the time you will not give a warning. If your child knows the rules and understands that when she hits her sister, she will go to time-out, no warning is necessary. Just place your child in time-out immediately when the misbehavior occurs.

2. Am I talking or arguing with my child before placing him in time-out or while he is serving time-out?
   The child should be ignored while in time-out, even if he is saying, "I like time-out. Leave me in time-out all day. I don't want to play anyway!" Remember to use no more than 10 seconds and 10 words to place your child in time-out.

3. Do I have an appropriate place for time-out?
   Remember, the location you select should be *dull* and nonreinforcing. Do not use your child's room. Select an area of the house that is away from the high-traffic area. Typically an uncomfortable, straight-back chair that is child size works well.

4. Am I keeping track of the time myself?
   It is advisable to use a portable timer. Place it within view but out of reach of your child. It helps if you obtain a timer that ticks loudly in order that your child can hear as well as see it. There are some children who are annoyed by the ticking sound of a timer, and their negative behavior escalates when the timer is heard. There are silent timers that use color to indicate the amount of time remaining in the time-out (Generaction, Inc., at 513-561-2599).

5. Do I occasionally threaten to use time-out and then not use it?
   Use time-out each time the selected misbehavior occurs. Threatening to use it will not decrease the behavior's occurrence rate. When you threaten to use time-out and then not use it, you increase the number of times the behavior occurs.

6. Do I have a set number of minutes my child will remain in time-out, or do I change the amount of time depending on the kind of day we are experiencing?
   Have a set amount of time for time-out. Use either 1 minute per year of age or a 5-minute time out. Select one of these and stick with it. It is fine to have a rule that if your child is not quiet when the timer rings, 1 minute will be added. It is also appropriate to inform your child that the time-out will not begin until she is quiet. If you use these approaches, be consistent.

7. Does my child understand when he will be sent to time-out?
   You should clearly explain to your child the behaviors for which he will be sent to time-out. Explain it to your child prior to the behavior's occurrence. Do this at a time when you and he are calm. It is beneficial for both parents to explain the time-out procedure. You may want to role-play a situation and the procedure that will be followed when this behavior is displayed. As you will recall, time-out should not be used for every misbehavior that occurs. It should be reserved for specific behaviors that warrant this type of punishment.

8. Are all caregivers using the same procedure for time-out?
   All adults who are responsible for disciplining your child should use the same procedure.

9. What do I do when the behavior occurs away from home?
   If possible, place the child in time-out at that location. If this is not possible or you do not feel comfortable with this, you may have a prearranged plan with your child that will inform your child that she will have to serve time-out immediately upon arriving home.

10. Is the remainder of the day pleasant for my child?
    Don't take your child's good behavior for granted. Remember to reinforce and praise your child for appropriate behavior the remainder of the day. Your child has served time-out, so there is no need to continue talking about the negative behavior the rest of the day. If time-out is more enjoyable than the time your child spends with you, time-out will not be an effective punishment.

mand. You will need to decide if the child will go to time-out the second or third time you give a command in which she or he did not comply. (Make sure the command is a good one; review Chapter 3). Initially, select one or two behaviors that will result in a time-out. The behavior must be countable (e.g., hitting sister, throwing toys).

Time-out is usually not effective in stopping behaviors such as whining, failing to complete chores or homework, overactive behaviors that are not aggressive but are just the result of the child's ADHD, being afraid or displaying other moods, behaviors that were not directly seen by you, not sharing with a sibling, or interrupting others' conversations.

2. *Select the place to be used for time-out.* This should be a dull setting where the child is not in danger of hurting himself or herself or others or destroying materials or property. Places parents have found effective for time-out include the hallway, a corner of a room, a bathroom, the wash room, or the corner of the porch. You may be able to identify other appropriate locations for time-out. It is not advisable to select your child's bedroom because many children have a television, a computer, games, and toys in the bedroom. Remember that time-out is a punishment. It should not be enjoyable. If you select the bathroom, child-proof it. As you will recall from the story at the beginning of this chapter, Matt's parents had failed to child-proof the bathroom prior to assigning him a time-out. Toilet paper is not dangerous. The child may unroll it, but she or he can roll it back when time-out is over.

3. *Count how often the misbehavior occurs.* You can do this by placing tally marks on a wall calendar. While this step is not imperative to using time-out, it is a good way to track the progress you are making and to discover if time-out is really working to decrease the inappropriate behaviors. If your child notices that you are counting the behaviors, just respond, "Your dad and I are concerned about the number of times you are sassy to us. I'm counting the number of times you are sassy. We are going to find a way to help you to stop this. I'll talk to you later about our plan." At times, this act of counting will reduce the number of times the inappropriate behavior occurs. Continue with the process anyway. When the novelty of your counting wears off, the behavior will reappear.

4. *Explain the time-out procedure to your child.* This explanation should occur prior to assigning the first time-out. It should be given at a time when everyone is in a good mood, not immediately after or during a confrontation with your child. If there are two parents in the home, both should be present. Don't argue or debate with your child; just present the facts: "Sarah, your mom and I have been concerned about the number of times you push and hit your sister. We want to help you to stop this because it is causing problems in our family. From now on, each time you hit or push your sister, your mom or I will say 'time-out.' That means that you must go to the chair in the laundry room and stay there for 5 minutes. If you don't go immediately or if you make a lot of noise getting there, you will have extra minutes added. Do you have any questions about time-out? Repeat back to me what you think time-out means and when you will be going." If Sarah does not appear to listen or fully understand these directions, give the explanation again. For young children, it is often helpful to role-play time-out using a doll.

5. *It is best to implement the time-out procedure on a day when both parents are at home in order that you can fully enforce the consequence.* Usually a Saturday morning works well. Don't try to use time-out, for the first time, on a day when you cannot devote full energy to it. If you are a single parent, ask a friend to help you by coming to your home on the morning you choose to begin time-out. Then just wait for the behavior to occur. If you have completed steps 1–4 as described above when the behavior occurs, you should have to do only two things: (1) label the misbehavior, and (2) state the consequence. It should take no more than 10 seconds and 10 words to do this. "That was backtalk. Go to time-out."

6. *There are several schools of thought on the amount of time a child should remain in time-out.* It has been demonstrated that a longer time-out is no more effective to stop misbehavior than a brief time-out. Thus, a parent could use the "1 minute per year of age" guideline or have a standard 5-minute time-out. Regardless of the time you select, keep the time consistent each time it is used. Do not make it 10 minutes one time because you are really angry or when your child is getting on your nerves.

A parent may have a rule such as, "If you are not quiet when the time-out ends (child is still screaming), one minute will be added until you are quiet for the last minute." Make sure this is agreed to by both parents and is followed consistently.

Occasionally, a parent asks, "What do I do when my child refuses to go to time-out?" This may happen the first few times you use time-out. If it does, you should not give in to your child. Escort your child (by a firm but not harsh approach) to the time-out area and insist that she or he remain in the chair or area and state that the time-out will not start until she or he is in the area without being restrained. After a few times, your child will learn that you are serious, and your child will not resist. However, you must stand firm and be consistent in your efforts or time-out will not work to stop an inappropriate behavior. This is the reason it was suggested to begin using time-out on a Saturday. It may take some time to train your child. If you give in to your child and let her or him out of time-out because of the screaming, your child has trained you to stop what she or he doesn't like (i.e., time-out) by screaming or being aggressive. Hang in there!

7. *Use a portable timer to keep track of the time.* Place the timer within view of your child but not where she or he can reach it to manipulate the time. This will prevent your child from asking, "How much time is left?" Do not try to keep track of the time yourself. You may get busy and forget what time you placed your child in time-out. This was the primary reason that time-out did not work for Matt. His dad failed to set the timer, and Matt remained in time-out beyond 5 minutes. This was enough time for a bright, inquisitive boy with ADHD to find something to do. Remember: do not give your child any attention or talk to your child while she or he is in time-out. Time-out is time away from reinforcement, negative or positive. Most parents use a portable timer that ticks loudly and can be heard from the time-out area. This type of timer works well with most children. A few children have responded better to a timer that is silent but visually displays the time remaining. These timers are named A Time Timer and are sold by Generaction, Inc., of Cincinnati, Ohio (513-561-2599).

8. *After the timer has rung, ask your child to state the reason for being in time-out.* You may do this step for children up to age 9 years. Use your own judgment when the child is older than 9. If after asking your child inappropriate behaviors escalate, do not ask the question at the end of the time.

9. *If your child was in time-out because of a failure to follow your command, re-issue the command immediately after the timer rings.* For example, "John, I need you to go to your room and pick up your toys." If he refuses to follow this command after it was given two times, instruct him to go to time-out. When he completes his 5-minute time-out, re-issue the command: "John, I need you to pick up your toys in your room." Wait 5 seconds. If he refuses, place him in another 5-minute time-out. Continue this process until he complies with your command. *Do not give in out of frustration.* This is one of the reasons for the friend or spouse being with you on the first day you use time-out. You will likely need support and encouragement to avoid giving in to your child.

One parent reported to me that she was putting a great deal of effort into consistently using appropriate punishment strategies with her son, but she was experiencing difficulty remembering the consequences she and her son had developed for each misbehavior or for rules that were not followed. When her child demonstrated his "sassy remarks to his sister," she was so upset with him that she could not quickly recall the specific punishment. To aid her memory, she and her son created a "Rule System Guide." When discussing the misbehavior with her son, who was 8 years of age, she wrote the misbehavior or rule on one side of an index card. On the reverse side, she recorded the consequence for this misbehavior. For example, when Travis made a sassy remark to his sister, the consequence for this misbehavior was that he was required to write 10 positive statements about her. She punched holes in the cards and secured these on one large metal key ring. Until the consequences were learned, she carried these cards with her everywhere. When Travis violated one of the rules, she handed him the cards, he read the reverse side, and he proceeded to follow through with the consequence.

Final Notes

Now that you have been introduced to a number of parenting suggestions, you may think your work as a parent will be easy. Parenting a child with ADHD requires better parenting skills than parenting the "easy" child. In the process of parenting these difficult children, you will develop a bond with this child that is often not present with the child that just raises herself or himself. Thus, there are some benefits to having a child who requires a great deal of attention and special parenting. Even with these strategies, Patterson and Forgatch (1987, pp. 164–168) suggest that it is important to remember a number of key factors in trying to change inappropriate behavior:

- *Behavior changes slowly.* Don't expect immediate changes in your child's behavior just because a punishment is used. It usually takes weeks to see major changes.

- *When you decide to use a certain punishment for a specific behavior, be consistent.* When you decide on a behavior to punish, punish it every time it occurs, not every third time or only when you are in a bad mood.

- *Long lectures do not change behavior.* If you give your child a lecture, she or he usually tunes you out after a few minutes. The lecture is often used by the parent to make the parent feel better, not to make the child behave better.

- *Punishment by itself is not enough to change behavior.* You must, at other times, demonstrate respect and love for your child and give her or him attention and generous amounts of positive feedback for appropriate behavior.

- *Punishment is more effective when it is delivered in a calm manner.* The louder and more emotional you become, the louder and more emotional your child's outbursts will likely be.

- *Mild forms of punishment are more effective than severe ones.*

Changing Behavior

> Many things we need can wait. The child cannot. Now is the time his bones
> are being formed; his blood is being made; his mind is being developed. To him
> we cannot say tomorrow. His name is today.
>
> —Gabriela Mistral

When parenting a child with disruptive behaviors, one quickly discovers that positive reinforcement is frequently not enough to motivate a child to follow the rules, comply with requests, or complete chores. Other parents, as well as some teachers, think that punishments should work to motivate a child. Recently, a teacher wrote a note on a child's referral form for testing: "I've tried taking away all kinds of privileges, but nothing seems to motivate her." As discussed in the previous chapter, punishments by themselves will not motivate a child to demonstrate appropriate behaviors. When positive reinforcements and punishments are not enough to replace an inappropriate behavior with an appropriate behavior, it becomes necessary to identify other methods to motivate the child.

What can I do to get my child more motivated to change her behaviors?

A behavior change program is one approach that has been helpful in motivating a child to replace inappropriate behaviors with appropriate ones. This type of program works well when one or two specific behaviors are becoming increasingly problematic and positive reinforcement has not worked to sufficiently motivate the child to change a behavior. Before developing a behavior change program, it is essential that you identify two things: (1) the problem behavior you want to weaken and (2) the opposite positive (pro-social) behavior you want to take its place. For example, the problem behavior may be your child's excessive number of times she or he "talks back" to you in a sassy tone of voice or the number of times she or he argues with you. The opposite pro-social behavior you want to take its place is complying with your request in a reasonable time period without a sassy comment or an argument.

As suggested in the last chapter, behaviors take time to change. Even with a punishment or a behavior change program, it will still take time to change negative behaviors that have become habits. Gerald Patterson (1975) has developed a series of steps that are useful in changing problem behaviors to positive pro-social behaviors. Below are the initial steps for a behavior change program (Patterson, 1975; and Patterson & Forgatch, 1987):

1. *Determine the behavior you want weakened (decreased), as well as the pro-social behavior you want to take its place (increased).* Pinpoint the specific behavior you want to

weaken. It should be observable and countable. If a parent says, "I want to change my child's immature behavior," this is not countable. The behavior must be specific enough that it can be counted. Ask yourself, "What about my child's behavior makes me describe it as immature?" You may respond, "She talks like a baby. She whines when she doesn't get her way. She throws a temper tantrum when she doesn't get her way." These behaviors are observable and countable. The first time you attempt this program, select a behavior that occurs at least 5 times each day. This will make it easier to observe changes and for both you and your child to see progress.

2. *Count the behaviors.* Count the behaviors for 3 or 4 days. While counting, do not use a program. (You do not have to count the behaviors in order to have change; however, counting the behavior helps determine the progress made, and occasionally counting a behavior actually may help to temporarily decrease its rate of occurrence.) A sample Tracking Card is shown in Figure 6.1, and a blank Tracking Card is in Appendix C. Use this form to track the number of times the behavior occurs and then determine the rate (average number of occurrences per hour). For example, if you counted 10 times in a 2-hour block of time that your child responded to you in a sassy tone of voice, the rate per hour would be 5 per hour. You do not need to count these behaviors 24 hours a day to obtain a rate. Select several times during the day to count the behaviors (e.g., between 5:00 P.M. and 7:00 P.M., between 6:00 A.M. and 7:00 A.M.).

3. *Establish a baseline.* Count the same behaviors on at least 2 other days in order to obtain an average number over 3 to 4 days. A child will typically have some good days and some bad. If you find that your child has all good days when you are counting, continue to count for several more days. Some parents find that it helps to graph the average occurrence rate per day; however, this is not necessary. Also, some parents have had their child graph the number of times the behavior occurs. Many children will deny that they have a problem, and by counting and graphing the behaviors, the child becomes more aware of the behaviors. The child's graphing of the behavior should occur after you have completed your 2 to 4 days

---

Behavior Tracking Card

Behavior to increase: <u>Using an appropriate tone of voice or complying with a command without a comment.</u>

Behavior to decrease: <u>Using a sassy tone of voice or arguing with Mom or Dad when a command or request is given.</u>

Behaviors	Day <u>Saturday</u> Time <u>1:00–3:00 P.M.</u>	Day <u>Sunday</u> Time <u>1:00–3:00 P.M.</u>	Day <u>Monday</u> Time <u>5:00–7:00 P.M.</u>	Day <u>Tuesday</u> Time <u>5:00–7:00 P.M.</u>
Behavior to increase	II Rate: <u>.5/hour</u>	IIII Rate: <u>2/hour</u>	II Rate: <u>1/hour</u>	II Rate: <u>1/hour</u>
<u>Appropriate tone of voice</u>				
Behavior to decrease	̶H̶H̶ I Rate: <u>3/hour</u>	̶H̶H̶ II Rate: <u>4/hour</u>	̶H̶H̶ Rate: <u>2.5/hour</u>	̶H̶H̶ I Rate: <u>3/hour</u>
<u>Sassy tone of voice or arguing</u>				

Rate for positive behavior: <u>1.25/hour</u>
Rate for inappropriate behavior: <u>3.125/hour</u>

FIGURE 6.1. Sample Tracking Card.

of counting. Graphing also helps some children become more aware of their improvement.

 ## How do I implement a behavior change program with my child?

After you have counted the behaviors, you are now ready to develop a program for change. *Contracts* usually work well in developing a program. It should be remembered that the older the children, the more involved they should be in developing the contract. With young children, the parent will develop most of the contract. The steps to developing a contract are listed below:

1. *Explain the idea to your child.*

DAD: Brandon, you have noticed that your mom and I have been counting the number of times you make sassy remarks to us. We don't like fussing at you for this. So we are going to help you with this problem. If you do as we request, without a sassy remark, you will earn 5 points each time. We will add these points to your chart.

BRANDON: What do I get for the points?

DAD: At the end of each day, we will count the points, and you can select something from the menu of rewards we are going to develop. What do you think a sassy remark is?

BRANDON: It's when I say a smart-mouth remark and don't do what you say.

DAD: Can you make a sassy remark without opening your mouth?

BRANDON: Yes, by giving you or Mom a mean look or rolling my eyes at you.

DAD: What can you do other than give a sassy remark?

BRANDON: Do what you say without saying anything or tell you okay.

DAD: Maybe you could say, "I got you covered" and this would be okay if you have to say something. I think you understand, but let's practice one time to see if you know what we expect. Let's think of some things you would like to earn with your points, and then we will sign the contract together. This will be fun.

Most children between the ages of 8 and 12 respond positively to the use of points in developing a behavior change program. With children younger than 8, it is often better to use something tangible, such as poker chips, marbles, or buttons, to represent the points. In addition, some older children who have a language disorder will also need to use a tangible reinforcer. With many children who are 12 and older, it will be necessary to negotiate a contract, and many may not respond well to points. You will need to develop the contract in such a way that the teen can earn or lose specified privileges depending on the behaviors demonstrated.

2. *Put the agreement in writing.* This could be done on the Weekly Point Chart (to be described later) or in a Written Agreement (as seen in Figure 6.2). Younger children or children with reading problems may need pictures rather than words. As progress is made, gradually increase the demands placed on your child to reach a goal. A blank form can be found in Appendix C.

3. *Develop a menu of rewards.* The parent and child should prepare a menu of rewards (see sample form in Figure 6.3 and a blank form in Appendix C). Some of the

---

Contract

I, Brandon, agree to do what Mom and Dad tell me to do without making a sassy remark. I can say "I got you covered" or "okay" when they tell me to do something, and that will not count as a sassy remark unless I use an ugly tone of voice when saying it.

We, Mom and Dad, agree to award Brandon with 5 points each time he uses an appropriate tone of voice and/or does what we say without saying anything. We will also make sure we give a "good command" and will be aware that sometimes Brandon is busy with a project, playing with his computer, or watching television and it may not be a good time to give a command. We will work hard to time our commands and to give them appropriately to avoid setting Brandon up for a failure. Sometimes, Brandon will understand that we must ask him to do something even though he is involved in something. We will allow Brandon to select a reward from his menu of rewards when he obtains enough points. We will be sure to follow through and give him the rewards.

Date contract begins: Saturday, March 7, 1998
Date contract is reevaluated: Saturday, March 14, 1998
Date contract ends or is renegotiated: April 15, 1998

_____   _____
Child's Signature   Date

_____   _____
Mother's Signature   Date

_____   _____
Dad's Signature   Date

FIGURE 6.2. Sample written agreement.

rewards should be small and obtainable on a daily basis, and others could be larger to encourage your child to save some daily points (chips) for a larger reward. Determine the number of points (chips) that are needed for each reward. During the first week that this program is used, it is important for the child to experience success; therefore, establish the point/chip system low enough in order that the child can reach at least one reward the first day.

4. *You and your child should sign the contract (or point sheet) and follow through with the agreement.* Do not abruptly stop the program, or the child's behavior will likely revert back to the original problem behaviors. Gradually wean your child from the rewards or gradually increase the demands on her or his behavior to earn a reward. During the first phase of this program, *do not* take away points or chips. If this does not result in gradual improvement in 2 to 3 weeks, evaluate the program for reasons it is not working. Possible reasons include the following:

> *The steps in the program were too large.* For example, are you requiring that your child clean her or his entire room, when the smaller steps of picking up the toys, making the bed, or putting dirty clothes away have not been mastered? You may need to break down the steps into "baby" steps for your child to be successful the first week. After she or he has reached a level of consistency with the "baby" steps, gradually require more from your child.

> *You failed to pair a social reinforcer (praise, hug, pat on the back) with the tangible reward (star, button, point, chip) each time you observed the pro-social behavior.*

> *You were not consistent with the program.* For example, one father overheard his child tell the baby-sitter when asked about the point chart on the bulletin board,

Menu of Rewards	
Menu of Privileges and Rewards	**Cost in Points/Chips**
1. Jump on trampoline with Mom or Dad.	15
2. Say up 1/2 hour later on a school night.	40
3. Control of the remote for 1/2 hour.	50
4. 15-minute backrub from mom or dad.	20
5. One less chore for next day.	40
6. Dinner in the family room.	50
7. Trip to the pet store.	50
8. Select the dessert for dinner.	60
9. Trip to McDonald's.	75
10. Bake cookies with Mom or Dad.	100

FIGURE 6.3. Sample menu of rewards.

"Yes, this is my point sheet, but Mom and Dad don't do it every day. So it doesn't matter if I follow it."

The family members did not follow the procedures as outlined in the contract for rewards and punishment.

The child does not appear to like the rewards. If the rewards are not powerful enough, the behavior will not change. Always involve the child in the selection of rewards.

The rewards were available to the child at other times. If they are available at other times and are not contingent on meeting the criteria set in your contract, you will not see changes in your child's behavior. These rewards need to be special and are earned only when the child reaches a goal. Select other rewards if these are not appropriate. For example, one mother had listed "Katherine can chew sugar-free gum when she obtains 15 points." This reward was not a good reward because Katherine was allowed to chew gum any time she wanted. If Katherine were only allowed to chew gum when she had earned 15 points, it is likely that this would have been a good motivator.

 ### *My child has more than one behavior that needs to change. Are there other ways that I can help him?*

A point system is another approach that works to decrease inappropriate behaviors and increase pro-social behaviors. A point system is essentially a contract that is in the form of a *checklist.* As mentioned previously, point systems are usually not effective with older children (12 years and older); negotiation and contract development have been found to be more effective with the adolescent. Patterson (1975) suggests several advantages to using a checklist:

1. You can simultaneously strengthen a number of behaviors that "occur sometimes but are still relatively weak and unpredictable" (p. 63).

2. It saves you from having a series of six or seven behavior change programs running simultaneously.

3. It can also extend to situations where you are not present (e.g., school, day-care, grandmother's house).

4. It is an excellent way to develop home–school collaboration because you can provide reinforcement for behaviors that occur at school.

The steps for establishing a point system are as follows:

1. *Select behaviors you want to improve.* You may have identified several behaviors in Chapter 2 that you want to see your child do more often. Select the behaviors you want to increase (e.g., making bed each morning, putting dirty clothes in the clothes hamper, brushing teeth before school, going to bed by 8:30 P.M. without an argument). Attempt to describe these behaviors in the positive rather than the negative. For example, rather than "Stop leaving toys in the living room," state it as "Pick up toys before going to bed."

2. *Make a point-reward chart.* List on the chart the behaviors you want your child to strengthen. Involve your child in this process. It is also wise to list the time you will check for completion of the behavior. Next to each behavior, indicate the number of points/chips the child will earn upon completion of the behavior. Post the chart. Children younger than 8 years will likely need chips or some other token reinforcer (e.g., beans, marbles, buttons, play money), rather than points. Because of their developmental level, they will need something concrete in order to know that they have earned the points. Figure 6.4 illustrates one point-reward chart that was developed by the parents of a 10-year-old. As you will note, some of the behaviors are more advanced than would be used if a child were just beginning to use a point system (e.g., Heather will be awake, be dressed, and be downstairs by 7:00 A.M.). A younger child would probably need this step broken down into three behaviors. You will also note that some behaviors earn more points. Heather experienced greater difficulty following the homework routine; thus, a higher point value was given to this behavior. (A blank Weekly Point Chart can be found in Appendix C.)

3. *Develop a menu of rewards.* For this point/chip system to work, it is critical that you identify the right rewards for your child. What may be a reward for me may not be for you. It is best to develop the reward list with your child (see sample in Figure 6.3 and a blank form in Appendix C). The rewards should be small enough that they can be earned daily; however, the parent may identify several larger rewards that will require that the child save points for several days. Try to include several activity rewards (e.g., playing basketball with mom) as well as a few tangible rewards (e.g., a movie to rent). It is necessary, at times, to tell your child when a reward is not appropriate. For example, when one father asked his son, "What would you like to earn if you have 25 points?" His son responded, "A trip to DisneyWorld." Dad responded, "I can't afford that, and it is too large of a reward for only 25 points. Think of some things that are small but those that you would like." The first time you develop a menu of rewards, you and your child may need to spend some time in a brainstorming session.

4. *Keep track of the points your child earns and spends (see blank form in Appendix C).* When checking to see that your child has earned points, record them on the chart and enthusiastically provide a social reinforcement (praise). If your child fails to earn the points for "making her bed by 7:00 A.M.," do not lecture. Just comment, "Heather, you didn't earn your points for making your bed by 7:00, but I'm sure you can do it tomorrow." Do not take away points for inappropriate behavior at this time. Use other forms of appropriate punishment for these behaviors. For example, you may have on the checklist that your child will have a back talk–free day. If the punishment for "talking back" is a 5-minute time-out, then place your child in time-out if she or he talks back. Reward the child with the appropriate number of points if she or he has a back

Weekly Point Chart

Behavior (points)	Mon.	Tues.	Wed.	Thurs.	Fri.	Sat.	Sun.
1. Heather will be awake, be dressed, and be downstairs by 7:00 A.M. (10)							
2. Ready to walk out the door by 7:30— backpack in hand, teeth brushed, and hair combed! (15)							
3. Adheres to assigned homework time. (25)							
4. 15 minutes of piano practice without complaining. (15)							
5. Pack backpack for next day. Place by back door, clothes laid out. (10)							
6. Bath taken, teeth brushed, and in bed by 8:00 P.M. (15)							
Total points earned							

Child's Signature   Date   Mother's Signature   Date

Father's Signature   Date

FIGURE 6.4. Sample point-reward chart.

talk–free day. (Note: If your child has many instances of talking back each day, a back talk–free day may be unattainable. Break it down into smaller steps. For example, a back talk–free morning before going to school, a back talk–free afternoon before dinner, and a back talk–free evening before going to bed. Then, as progress is made, you can increase the time to a back talk–free day.)

5. *Modify the point chart as needed.* After using the point system for a while, you may discover that clearer definitions for behaviors need to be made, that rewards need to be changed, or that behaviors need to be broken down into smaller steps. Review the old charts and evaluate the progress made. If one behavior is particularly difficult for your

child, award more points for that behavior than for others, or you may break it down into smaller steps.

One good technique to keep the motivation high is to provide a "mystery motivator" for meeting all goals for a given day. A "mystery motivator" as described by William Jenson (1995) from the University of Utah is prepared in the following way: Prepare an envelope with a question mark (?) on the front. Inside, write a reward that your child can earn if the goal is reached. The reward can be one that is earned for the entire family or for your child alone, such as taking the entire family to a fun restaurant, no chores for one day, or going fishing after school. If the child reaches the prearranged goal, she or he earns the right to open the envelope and receive the reward. If your child does not reach the goal, the envelope remains sealed and can be earned another day. Mystery motivators are often helpful when a point system has been in place for some time and a new motivator is needed to increase the interest level for your child.

6. *Gradually phase out the point chart.* If your child's behavior has improved to the point that a structured program is no longer needed, phase it out. This needs to be done gradually. This can be accomplished by increasing the number of days a behavior must occur before points are awarded (e.g., earning points for making the bed for an entire week rather than 2 consecutive days). Continue to praise the positive behavior. This, however, can also be gradually reduced to periodic praising. Occasional praise will *always* be needed. You may consider having a "graduation party," informing your child, "You have improved and are doing so well, let's have a party to celebrate because you no longer need a point chart."

Final Notes

Based on the information presented in this chapter, you should decide if a point/chip checklist or a behavior change program is needed for your child. If you have several behaviors to increase, a point system will work if your child is younger than 12 years, and a contract will usually work well for the individual who is 12 and older. If you have one inappropriate behavior you want to replace with an opposite positive behavior, a behavior change program can work. Do not attempt to implement both simultaneously. Choose one and develop a program at home from start to finish with your child.

Building Self-Esteem in Your Child

Children will not remember you for the material things you
provided but for the feeling that you cherished them.

—Richard L. Evans

Many parents of children with ADHD report concern that their children appear to have poor self-esteem. When individuals have healthy self-esteem, they can meet the challenges of life with confidence in their ability to master them successfully (Chess & Thomas, 1987, p. 155). When children receive frequent negative remarks or numerous verbal reprimands from teachers, peers, and parents, they usually regard themselves as having low worth, and they feel inadequate to meet the demands placed on them. Although these interactions with others are not the sole reason for poor self-esteem, they do contribute to the children's overall view of themselves. Approaches to enhance your child's self-worth will be presented in this chapter, with most of the information presented being a review of the previous five chapters. As you will probably quickly observe, the enhancement of a person's self-worth generally improves when the principles of social learning included in this book are practiced.

What is self-esteem?

Dorothy Corkille Briggs (1975, p. 3) defines self-esteem as "how a person feels about himself. It is the overall judgment of himself; how much he likes his particular person." Robert Brooks (1991, p. 3) notes that some individuals define self-esteem as the difference between a person's "ideal self" (how one would like to be) versus how the person actually perceives herself or himself. The larger the gap between the two, the lower the person's self-esteem. Robert Brooks (1992, p. 538) suggests that we look beyond these definitions that focus primarily on a person's "feelings" or how one "thinks" because of the "confusion between self-esteem and self-centeredness, conceit, and selfishness." In 1988 the California Task Force to Promote Self-Esteem and Personal and Social Responsibility included the following as part of the definition of self-esteem: "appreciating my own worth and importance . . . but having the character to be accountable for myself and to act responsibly toward others" (Brooks, 1991, p. 3). In other words, Brooks suggests that to have positive self-esteem, a person will be acting responsibly toward others, as well as being accountable for her or his own actions.

My adult children can probably still hear me saying each of the following statements at some time when they were younger: "You are responsible for your own actions." "The fact that you have ADHD or are upset because you feel that someone mistreated you does not change who you are as a person." Another comment they frequently heard was, "The other person didn't *make* you act this way or *make* you mad. You made the decision to respond the way you did."

❓ *How can I know if my child has poor self-esteem?*

One of the characteristics often seen in children who have inadequate self-esteem is that they blame their situations on others or their "dumb luck"—"someone made me do it." In other words, they are attributing their success or failure to something out of their control. Thus, it is difficult for them to assume responsibility for their actions. Bernard Weiner (as quoted by Reid & Borkowski, 1987) refers to this as the *Attribution Theory*. To what does your child attribute her or his success or failure? Many children who have ADHD or a learning disability frequently attribute their success or failure to situations outside their control. For example, a child who does poorly on a test might respond, "The teacher doesn't like me. He gives stupid tests. He didn't tell us to study that." Comments such as these are likely a reflection of a child's poor self-esteem. A child who attributes success or failure to her or his own efforts might respond, "Next time, I'll study harder. I forgot to study that part." It is also not uncommon for children who have low self-esteem to make comments such as the following even when they do well: "I was lucky. She asked easy questions" (Reid & Borkowski, 1987).

❓ *How can I help my child begin to assume more responsibility for what happens to her?*

You can help your child in the process of learning to attribute success or failure to her or his own efforts by discussing these comments and by asking questions such as, "What could you do next time to do better on the test?" Help your child generate ideas if none come to mind. For example, you might suggest that she or he talk to the teacher before the test to determine what needs to be studied or ask her or his parents for help when studying. Also, avoid overreacting when your child does poorly. Your overreaction may result in your child feeling that an excuse for failure is needed, rather than using it as an opportunity to learn from the failure. It can also be helpful if you model an appropriate response when you make a mistake or experience a failure. For example, if you were not successful at something at work, you might respond, "Boy, I goofed at work today because I didn't listen to what my boss said." You are demonstrating to your child that you are assuming responsibility for your own mistakes or failures.

Ted Engstrom, in his book *The Pursuit of Excellence* (1982), discusses how some very successful people have succeeded despite their failures. He details the life of Abraham Lincoln prior to being elected president of the United States in 1860:

> He grew up on an isolated farm and had only one year of formal education. In those early years, he was exposed to barely half a dozen books. In 1832 he lost his job and was defeated in the race for the Illinois legislature. In 1833 he failed in business. In 1834 he was elected to the state legislature, but in 1835 his sweetheart died, and in 1836 he had a nervous breakdown. In 1838 he was defeated for Speaker of the House, and in 1843 he was defeated for nomination for Congress. In 1846 he was elected to Congress but in 1848 he was rejected for a federal land officer appointment, and in 1854 he was defeated for the Senate. In 1856 he was defeated for the nomination of vice president, and in 1858 he was again defeated for the Senate. (pp. 76–77)

When children experience failure in their lives, do not imply that they will be failures throughout their lives. With your encouragement to take each failure or mistake and to gain insight into what can be learned from the experience, your child can emerge as a sensitive and successful person of worth and value. A mistake or failure does not make your child a failure. Children's experiences of failure may really be opportunities for success that have yet to be discovered.

[?] *What other factors contribute to my child's feelings of self-worth?*

Brooks (1991) emphasizes the importance of empathy and seeing "the world more clearly through the eyes" (p. 16) of the children if one is to discover the factors that are significant in raising children and to understand the role of self-esteem in a person's life. A difficult task, but one that can be helpful in the acquisition of empathy, is "to describe a typical day in your child's life, but through your child's eyes" (p. 17). In the space below, describe a typical day in your child's life, but through your child's eyes. Begin with the morning routine and really listen to what you say to your child each morning. Do your comments and actions tell your child that you think she or he is competent, even if there has been a failure or a mistake? Does she or he have responsibilities that encourage and foster positive self-worth?

_____

_____

_____

_____

_____

_____

_____

_____

Think of two experiences you have had in which one resulted in success and the other in failure. What factors do you believe contributed to the two outcomes? Now think of an experience that you initially viewed as a failure but you were able to turn around to be a stepping stone to a later success. While parents play an important role in the way in which children handle success and failure, and subsequently the way they view their self-worth, teachers will also affect the children. Recently, the importance of the teacher in the role of self-esteem building was made evident.

▶ The parents of a 10-year-old boy recently brought him to our clinic. He had participated in our summer treatment program the previous summer. He had made excellent progress in his behavior; however, he continued to struggle academically. Josh had actually done quite well until the middle of the school year. His parents had moved to a farm, and Josh was in his third school for that year. Josh's behavior had worsened at school, as well as at home. After a difficult day at school, Josh usually handled his frustration by being aggressive to his mother and siblings. After speaking with Josh's father for some time, his father shared with me three pages of handwritten notes that had been taken at school. In an attempt to help Josh improve his behavior in the classroom, his teacher had informed the child who was seated next to Josh to write on the paper each time Josh exhibited an inappropriate behavior. These are only a few of the more than 50 statements written in two days:

8:54   Josh said, "This is stupid."

8:55   Josh made a poot sound.

9:01   Josh yelled out loud.

9:07   Josh talked without permission (with 37 tics)

9:18   Josh made hissing sounds (3 tics)

11:10   He said he had "suicidal soup" for breakfast.

11:44   He got behind the teacher and danced.

12:38   Josh ran to his desk.

12:39   Josh laughed out loud.

12:56   He yelled, "No!"

  1:50   He took his hand off his mouth and talked.

These comments continued for three pages. The following was the last entry on day three:

  9:45   He made a face at the teacher when she told him to go in the hall and when she told him he said, "Thank you, Lord!"

After reading these entries, the teacher felt that Josh needed to be out of that classroom. The teacher's solution to the problem was possibly one of the worst examples of problem solving ever recorded in a school. Think for a minute through the eyes of Josh. Would this approach positively or negatively affect Josh's behavior? Remember that ridicule and sarcasm do not result in improved behavior. If Josh is like most of us, this approach would have increased the rate with which negative behaviors were occurring. Josh was in a negative cycle, and he saw no way out. After I spoke to Josh, the severity of his condition was apparent. He was referred for immediate psychiatric intervention. Of course, the episode with the teacher did not cause all the problems, but it did demonstrate the fragile nature of some of our children. We assume that because a child "acts tough," he must be able to handle harsh, severe consequences. If the teacher had wanted to use a student to help Josh improve his behavior, why not suggest to the peer to write an entry each time Josh demonstrated an appropriate behavior? When five appropriate behaviors were listed, the peer and Josh could earn a special reward. This likely would have improved Josh's behavior.

The principles and strategies presented in this book are also helpful in cultivating and fostering self-esteem in your child or adolescent. These principles, along with additional ideas, are presented below:

▶ Cultivate respect for your child.

• Since parents and other caregivers are the child's first mirrors, your attention and words have enormous weight.

• Demonstrate that you respect your child. Never embarrass or insult your child in public or in the presence of her or his friends. Many parents treat their friends better than they do their children. Treat your child as you would like to be treated.

• Regardless of how severe the behavior, don't label your child a "troublemaker," a "bad child," or a "failure."

• Appreciate your child's individuality and develop an understanding of her or his temperament. Your child may not be like his or her "easy temperament" sister or "sweet little cousin" who never does anything wrong, but your child does have attributes to be appreciated. Enjoy your child's playfulness and energy. Keep a log of all the funny things your child does and says. You will have many more memories of your child's early years than the parents of the "sweet little cousin."

• Treat your children differently according to their differing needs. "Fair" and "equal" treatments are not the same.

▶ Locate and cultivate competencies in your child.

- One approach to heighten self-esteem is to provide your child with opportunities to develop many skills (e.g., swimming, gymnastics, music, scouts, Tae Kwon Do). Between the ages of 5 and 12, children are in the job of building skills. The more skills they acquire, the greater their self-worth and the more responsible they can be for their actions.

- Many children with ADHD experience difficulty sticking with an activity. Quite often, once the novelty wears off, the child is ready for a new activity. Develop strategies to motivate your child in an activity to reach a certain level of proficiency. For example, develop a contract with your child when she or he wants to begin guitar lessons. The contract might read that the child would agree to practice 15 minutes 5 days each week and continue with the lessons for 6 months. After 6 months, the two of you will decide whether lessons should be continued. Identify a consequence to be listed in the contract if the agreement is broken. Successfully fulfilling a contract and reaching mastery of a new skill will also heighten your child's self-worth.

- An individual's self-esteem may vary from one situation to another depending on the competencies needed in an activity. This will occur if your total self-worth is based on how you feel rather than the components suggested by Bob Brooks. Remember that learning from mistakes and failures can also heighten feelings of competence.

- Locate at least one competency in your child. This can serve as a catalyst for the development of others (Brooks, 1991).

- Let your children do for themselves what they are capable of doing. Too often, we do things for our children that they are fully capable of doing for themselves (e.g., make bed, clear table after dinner). Often parents say, "Oh, he'll just make a mess. It's easier if I just do it myself." If you do everything for your child, your child will lose many opportunities to build competencies.

- Encourage your child to stretch in many directions. You may need to break a big goal into "baby" steps for your child to gain new skills. For example, your child might not be ready to play on a baseball team, but you can provide him or her with opportunities that will build skills to reach a long-range goal of playing on a team.

- Don't be a servant to your child. This does not help your child to build and stretch in many directions.

▶ A parent's self-esteem is a significant variable in determining the environment created in the home.

- Take steps to improve your own feelings of self-worth if you feel you have low self-esteem. Many parents find that counseling helps in this area. Identify areas in which you can be successful or can begin to stretch in new directions.

- How difficult or easy your child is to parent may affect your feelings of self-worth. Some children come into the world with difficult temperaments. They cry frequently as infants, and parents find it difficult to please them during their toddler and young-child years. Often, the parent equates this "difficult temperament" as an inability to be a good parent. At times, grandparents, teachers, or other significant adults inform you on ways to raise your child and what you are doing wrong. This is particularly evident for the parent who is single. Single parents should identify a support system to help them in the parenting of their child with ADHD.

▶ Realize the importance of positive feedback and encouragement.

• Let your child know when you appreciate things that she or he has done or said. Be specific when giving this feedback. "It really makes me feel good when you tell me you love me." Many times we forget all about it when our child complies with a rule or request. This is a great time to give positive feedback.

• Commend your child for her or his efforts as well as for accomplishments (especially when it may be unexpected). All too often, we praise the *product* and fail to praise the *effort*. Many children with ADHD need the encouragement to continue to try, even when the outcome may not be perfect.

• Become an observer of yourself when reacting to your child's behavior. View what is happening in a situation the way a video camera would capture it. Occasionally, it may help to leave a cassette recorder on during a difficult time to determine the parents' role in the problem. For example, if getting your child to do homework is extremely frustrating, place the cassette recorder in a location that will capture on tape what is happening. Listen to it after your child has gone to bed and assess your own behavior and what you can change to make the situation more pleasant for your child.

• Practice "catching" your child when she or he is behaving appropriately. Look for opportunities to provide specific praise. For example, if your son and his sister are playing quietly together while you are on the phone, pause in the conversation and give them specific praise. Don't be afraid that good behavior will stop if you praise it.

• Tell a person other than your child something positive about your child. Say this in order that your child can hear you make the positive statement.

▶ Give focused attention to your child.

• Implement the "special time" procedure in your home if you haven't already started it (see Chapter 2).

• "Giving things" and "doing things" are no substitute for giving one's time and self. Many busy parents feel guilty because they do not have enough time to be with their children. In order to assuage these feelings of guilt, a parent will buy the child "things." Children would rather have the parents' time. They need more than quality time, they also need *more* of our time.

▶ Provide security and structure for children.

• Children need clearly defined rules for behavior and consistent consequences for misbehavior. Have you written your "house rules"? House rules will change as the child grows and matures or when a rule is no longer necessary because it is no longer a problem within the home.

• As children reach preadolescence or adolescence, they continue to need the security provided by structure and routines; however, the parent should become less authoritative and involve the adolescent in the development of this structure.

• As responsibility is demonstrated, the parent should gradually move toward giving the child more freedom. The key to making this work is to take "baby steps" to this end.

▶ Help your child to feel an increasing sense of ownership and responsibility for her or his behavior, actions, and education.

• Develop the habit of holding a "family council" when issues and problems need to be discussed. This is a good time to teach children how to solve problems in an effective way. One approach to teaching problem solving is the STPDE plan (see the sample in Figure 7.1 and see Appendix C for the worksheet):

Stop: What's the problem?

Think of as many solutions as possible for the problem (brainstorm).

Pick the best plan.

Do it!

Evaluate it. Did it work? If not, modify or pick another plan.

When you are first using this model for problem solving, work together with your children. First, help your children specifically determine the problem (S). This is often very difficult for children and sometimes even for adults. If it is a family problem, the family should discuss it together in a family council format. If the problem is between two members of the family or with a peer, the two, with the parent, should work through these steps until the children are able to use this approach on their own. As the children become more proficient in solving problems, the parent should stay out of the problem-solving session. Let the children practice solving their own problems.

Problem-Solving Worksheet

1. **S**TOP: What is the problem?
   Our family never seems to have any "fun" time together because Mother is always working around the house.

2. **T**HINK of as many plans as possible that might help to solve the problem.

   1. Ask Grandmother to help with the chores.   2. Hire a maid to help with the chores.
   3. Let the girls clean the house.   4. Let's divide the chores among all of us.

3. **P**ICK the best plan.
   1. Grandmother can't help because she lives too far away. This solution won't work.
   2. We don't have enough money to hire a maid. This idea would not work.
   3. Cleaning the house is not just a girl's job. While Thomas liked this idea (he suggested it), Mother vetoed this solution.
   4. The family decided that Solution 4 was the best solution because it would not cost any money, it was fair to everyone, and it would get everyone involved. The family made a list of all the chores that needed to be completed on a daily and/or weekly basis. Each member of the family selected a chore until all the chores had been selected. Each child selected chores on his or her ability level. Emily thought it would be a good idea to make a chart. She completed this task.

4. **D**O the plan.

5. **E**VALUATE the plan. Was it a good plan? _X_ Yes ___ No
   How did it work?
   This solution worked extremely well for 2 months. During the 3rd month, Mother discovered that Thomas was paying Emily to do his chores. This new problem was brought to the group and the process began again.

FIGURE 7.1. Sample STPDE plan.

The second step of the STPDE plan is to brainstorm for possible solutions (T). When brainstorming, no response should be criticized. One person should put in writing all the suggestions, regardless of how ridiculous some may be.

In step 3, the family will select the best plan (P). Each idea suggested in the brainstorming session will be discussed. What is good about this idea, what is bad, why won't this work in our family, why will this work in our family? The family will select the plan that they perceive is the best one. This works best when the family can come to a consensus on the solution to select. Occasionally, you may allow your children to select a plan that may not be the best one. This can be a learning experience also.

In step 4, the plan is put into action (D). If this is a group problem-solving session, it is usually advisable to put the plan in writing and have all those present sign the plan.

In step 5, decide on a time to revisit the plan to determine how it is working and if any changes need to be made in the plan (E).

▶ As a single-parent family, we often used the family council to solve our problems. Any member of the family was permitted to present a problem for discussion. In one session, a problem was presented by me. The problem: There were so many jobs to do around the house that I felt that we never had time to just play or enjoy each other's company. I was working full time as well as working toward my doctorate at the time. After the problem was presented, each child presented a number of ideas in the brainstorming session. Thomas contributed that he thought we should get a maid to help with the work. Emily thought we could have grandmother help us. After a number of other ideas, the family decided that the best plan was to make a list of all the jobs that needed to be completed each week. After the jobs were listed, each person would select a job until all the jobs were selected. While the jobs were selected based on the person's developmental level, we all had specific jobs for which we alone were responsible. The agreement was put in writing, and we all signed it. We agreed to meet again the next week to see how the plan was working. The plan actually worked quite well for 2 months before a problem occurred. Thomas had gotten tired of his jobs and had persuaded Emily to complete his jobs for money. This resulted in another problem-solving session, which generated another solution.

Below you will find another contract that was written between Thomas and me as a result of problems associated with driving.

▶ Thomas can use his car on weekdays and weeknights to go to school, church, or school-related activities; however, he must be home by 10:00 P.M. when he has school the next day. On weekends or when he does not have school the following day, he can stay out until midnight. Thomas agrees to pay for gas and any traffic tickets he receives while using the car. He will not allow any other person to drive the car without his mother's permission. If the car's tires wear out within 18 months of purchasing them, he agrees to purchase new ones. He understands that he cannot drive the car when the tires are in poor condition.

Thomas also agrees to spend 45 minutes each school night sitting at his study desk. (This time can be divided into two study sessions totaling 45 minutes.) If he does not sit at his desk for 45 minutes each school night, he agrees to have the car home early for the number of minutes he did not study. If he fails to arrive home at the designated time, he will lose the car for one day for each 15-minute block of time he is late. For example, if he is

30 minutes late one night, he will not have the car for 2 days. If he is 1 hour late, he will not have the car for 4 days.

Thomas agrees that he will not drink and drive. If he is somewhere and has been drinking, he will call his mother. She will pick him up and ask no questions. If this becomes a habit, a new contract will be written to address this problem. If Thomas does drive after he has been drinking alcohol, his license will be taken away for 7 days, and he will not be allowed to drive during that time. He will also be required to come home immediately after school for 1 week and cannot go out on school nights or on the weekend for 1 week.

_____
Mother's Signature

_____
Thomas's Signature

_____
Date

- Let children solve some of their own problems and learn from their mistakes. Mistakes are to be learned from, not feel defeated by (Brooks, 1991). My 24-year-old son recently shared with me what he liked about my parenting style. He said that he liked it because I allowed the children to live their own lives, make some mistakes, learn from them, and then I was there to support and encourage them. What a relief! I had been feeling guilty that I had not prevented some of those mistakes.

- Don't bail your child out of every bad situation. Let your child suffer the natural consequence of an action if the situation is not harmful or dangerous. One parent shared with me her experience with her young adolescent son:

▶ A juvenile court officer called her at work late one afternoon. Her son had been brought there for shoplifting a compact disc. The parent was heartbroken. She couldn't believe he had done this. All the way to juvenile court, she cried, and then she knew what she must do. Since this was the first time her son had gotten into trouble, she thought the courts would probably just frighten him but let him go. To my surprise, she did not want this. She wanted her son to suffer the consequence of his action. She called an attorney friend, and it was decided that he would appear before the court and receive his consequence. He was fined $25 and 25 hours of public service work (picking up trash on the side of the road on 3 Saturdays).

While this was extremely difficult for this parent to do, the lesson learned from this mistake had long-lasting effects for her son. How many of you would allow your son to suffer the consequences of his actions? What better way to learn responsibility?

- As your children get older, let them set some of the rules for themselves, or at least allow them the opportunity to voice their opinions on the rules. Negotiate rules calmly. Of course, there are some rules that are nonnegotiable (e.g., no drinking while driving, no parties in the house without permission from a parent).

- Help your children set goals for themselves and provide them with encouragement to reach these goals.

▶ Create a sense of belonging for your child.

- Establish appropriate rituals and routines for your family (e.g., greetings and leave-takings, meals, bedtime). If you live in a busy household where both parents work, rituals and routines are even more important. One father developed the routine of spending the first 15 minutes after arriving home from work with his son. He gave his son focused attention for this time period, and he found that his son's behavior was better for the remainder of the evening. Why do you think his son's behavior would improve?

- Some chores should be assigned to each child in the family based on the child's age and abilities. Some chores should be assigned just because your child is a member of the family (e.g., putting clothes in the dirty clothes hamper), and there should be no payment for completing these chores.

- Make videotapes of special occasions to save and play later for friends and relatives.

- Give each child a bulletin board to be hung in a conspicuous place where she or he can put pictures, papers, articles, and the like. Leave it to your child to decorate and change as she or he desires.

- Give your child a private place of her or his own (e.g., own room or a portion of a room) where private possessions can be kept.

Final Notes

The principles presented thus far will have an impact on the establishment of your child's self-esteem. Although a single incident will not damage your child's self-esteem, a cycle of these negative events can result in poor self-esteem. You can help to promote a positive cycle by

- praising your child genuinely, especially when your child acts responsibly;

- giving of yourself and not just things;

- allowing your child to solve problems independently;

- allowing your child a voice in family decisions;

- giving physical affection and verbal affirmation;

- setting limits and providing structure when your child is young and allowing an older child to negotiate some privileges (Hannah & Stafford, 1993, p. 64).

The Home–School Connection

Keep away from people who try to belittle your ambitions. Small people always do that, but the really great make you feel that you, too, can become great.

—Mark Twain

▶ Joey, a fourth-grade student, is experiencing problems completing his classroom assignments during the school day. At home he does his homework, but he never seems to make it to school with homework in hand. There's always some excuse: "The dog ate it," "It's in my backpack, but I can't find it," or "Mom forgot to put it in my backpack." It isn't that Joey is rebelling against the system; it's just that he experiences significant problems with organization, or his mind wanders and he forgets what he was asked to do. Joey, like many other children with ADHD, needs his parents and teachers to provide external structure to assist with these problems. Joey's parents and his teacher have decided to develop a plan to address these concerns.

The connection between the home and the school is an important one. For children like Joey, a communication plan is needed whereby his parents and teachers view themselves as equal partners in educating Joey. Their roles may be different, but both must support the efforts of the other for Joey to benefit. In all situations (home and school), it is easier to prevent problems than to correct them after behaviors become problems. You may find, like many other parents, that your child experiences significant problems with school-related tasks. Some children with ADHD do fine academically, but many have learning problems. In a research project completed by Wolraich, Hannah, Pinnock, Baumgaertel, and Brown (1996), teachers of children in kindergarten through the fifth grade reported that of the children who met the DSM-IV criteria for ADHD, predominantly inattentive type, 72% were reported to have academic difficulties and only 33% had behavior problems. In contrast, of those children who were rated by their teachers to meet the criteria for the predominantly hyperactive/impulsive type, only 24% were reported to have academic problems, and approximately 73% were rated as having problems with behavior.

Regardless of the subtype of ADHD, children with this diagnosis will likely experience some type of school-related problem at some time in their school years. To intervene appropriately, it is necessary to apply the principles presented in this book. Although the problems may not be eliminated, they can be better managed.

❓ *Is there anything I can do to ensure that my child will be successful in school?*

Because reading is so crucial to individuals' success in their occupations, all parents of children with ADHD should first ensure that their children have acquired adequate basic reading skills. You may know that these skills are inferior by just listening to your child read. Other "at risk" factors include the following:

- family history of reading problems

- difficulty learning phonics

- history of articulation problems

- difficulty naming the letters of the alphabet

- word-finding problems

- mis-sequencing syllables when speaking (e.g., "aminals" for "animals")

- difficulty remembering verbal sequences (e.g., days of the week, months of the year in the correct order)

- difficulty remembering nursery rhymes as a preschooler

- problems in spelling as the child progresses through school

If your child reads poorly, and she or he also has a number of the "at risk" factors listed above, ask the school psychologist to evaluate your child for a possible learning disability or ask for additional help in reading. If you have the financial resources, a tutor can also assist your child with reading problems.

Second, proceed with caution when a teacher recommends that your child repeat a grade. Bachman, Green, and Wirtanen (1971) reported that students who were held back one grade increased the likelihood that they would drop out of school before graduation by 40% to 50%. This same study reported further that for students who were two grades behind, the risk of dropping out of school increased by 90% (Roderick, 1995). *Retention has not been demonstrated to be an effective remediation strategy.* If your child is not working on grade level, appropriate remediation strategies should be implemented, and retention should not be considered as the only remediation strategy. Giving a child "more of the same" will usually only delay academic problems, not eliminate them. Since children with ADHD attend better when the situation is novel, repeating a grade could result in greater problems with behavior and attention.

There are a number of academic areas that may be difficult for the child with ADHD. Below are the most common areas that impact the child with ADHD in the school setting, with suggestions for assisting the child who experiences these difficulties.

- *Written language:* This may be due to a child's poor fine motor skills or to other factors, such as a difficulty simultaneously attending to all the aspects of written language (punctuation, capitalization, vocabulary, grammar, spelling), a difficulty following multiple or sequential steps as in spelling, or viewing writing as a boring and repetitive task. The child with ADHD often does better when tasks are "new, novel, and exciting," and written language is often viewed by the child as the opposite of excitement. Allowing a child to use the word processor for long assignments has proved beneficial to many.

- *Taking notes:* Many children with ADHD will need specific instruction in note taking. As teens, they often report that they cannot listen and take notes at the same time. There are several strategies that can assist the adolescent in learning to take notes. One is to ask the teacher to provide an outline of the lecture to be presented. The teen could fill in the outline with the information presented in the lecture. Another approach would be to allow the teen to listen to the lecture and then borrow a peer's notes for studying. A common recommendation is to suggest that the student record the lecture. This is not always a good approach for the student with ADHD. First, if the student experiences difficulty remembering where she or he placed homework, how can the student be expected to remember to take the cassette recorder to class, remember to turn it on, remember to take it home, and then, if he or she does get it home, actually listen to it?

- *Rote memorization tasks:* Memorization requires sustained attention to a task that is frequently boring. Zentall and Gohs (1984) reported that children with ADHD tend to process global information better than they are able to process detailed information. Thus, the details of learning math facts or recalling specific information for which the child cannot attach meaning can be problematic. Interesting and stimulating computer software may be of assistance in learning the math facts.

- *Variability of performance:* Variability may appear in grades earned for one grading period or from day to day. This variability in performance is just part of the disorder. It is not clear why this inconsistency occurs in the child with ADHD. Russell Barkley (1995) suggests that in order for a person to produce consistent work, he or she must "inhibit impulses to engage in other, more immediately fun or rewarding activities, so the more limited and erratic one's impulse control, the more variable will be his or her work productivity" (p. 41). In other words, "productivity will depend more on the circumstances of the immediate situation than being dependent on self-control and willpower" (p. 41). If this is the case, then greater consistency will likely occur when the child or the adult who is working with the child can identify a motivator that is powerful enough to inhibit the impulsive responding.

- *Completion of assignments:* At times, this difficulty may be attributable to a problem in following multiple directions. At other times, it may be that the child becomes bored with the assignment and seeks stimulation from something else. Zentall and Meyer (1987) found that children with ADHD tend to perform best when presented with high-stimulation tasks that permit an active response. Since these children tend to be "seekers of stimulation" (as described by Zentall), they often experience difficulty completing repetitive tasks. Placing children in study carrels (cubicles) has not been demonstrated to result in increased attention and concentration (Ross & Ross, 1976), but this approach to reducing off-task behaviors continues to be widely used in many schools. Abramowitz and O'Leary (1991) did demonstrate, however, that when children worked at desks that were placed in rows, less off-task behavior and greater productivity during independent work were accomplished. Allowing the student to take a "stretch break" or to run an errand for the teacher seems to work well for some.

- *Organizational and study skills:* Many children with ADHD have significant problems getting and staying organized. Materials and books are lost, assignments are lost or not turned in even when completed, and papers are frequently messy and illegible. Most of these students need instruction and guidance in these areas. (Specific suggestions to address these concerns are presented in the next section of this chapter.)

- *Setting long-range goals:* Most children with ADHD have difficulty breaking a large task into smaller steps in order to complete it. Again, assistance will be needed to address this weakness.

• *Reading comprehension:* Some children with ADHD experience problems in understanding what they have read. This can occur even if the child does not have a learning disability. The child with ADHD may report, "I have to keep reading it over and over because I'll be reading along fine and then I get distracted by something else."

❓ What is the school's role in educating the child with ADHD?

Most schools now follow the steps described below when a child is experiencing problems with inattention or behavior, even when there has not been a formal diagnosis of ADHD.

▶ Step 1: In most schools, a "support team" (this team goes by different names in each system or state) is convened to address concerns expressed by parents or teachers.

This support team is a regular education function (as opposed to special education) and may include the principal, guidance counselor, classroom teacher(s), special educator, and occasionally the parent. Usually the support team meets weekly to discuss specific children who are experiencing academic, behavioral, or social problems. Parents are not always present at these meetings.

The support team will suggest interventions that the classroom teacher and parents can implement before a formal assessment is recommended or while the assessment is being completed. Occasionally, it is discovered that a child already has a diagnosis of ADHD. If so, a 504 plan may be developed. Section 504 of the Rehabilitation Act of 1973 is a civil rights law and prohibits discrimination against otherwise qualified persons with disabilities in federally assisted programs and activities solely on the basis of such person's disability. Under 504, the child's education must be provided in the regular education classroom unless it is demonstrated that education in the regular environment with the use of supplementary aids and services cannot be achieved satisfactorily.

There is more to helping children achieve than providing them with positive reinforcement and mild forms of consequences. Yes, these are important and necessary in any classroom, but these are reactive strategies—giving positive feedback or a consequence *after* a certain behavior occurs. To develop a balanced plan, the support team should consider proactive strategies that can be instrumental in preventing problems. The proactive strategies may be enough to solve some of the behavioral or attentional problems. If they are not enough for some children, the reactive strategies, such as an individualized behavior change plan, may be needed.

It is helpful if you, as the parent, know how to effectively advocate for your child. When advocating for your child, it is appropriate to be assertive but not aggressive in interactions with school personnel. The older children get, the more they should be able to advocate for themselves. By the time adolescents are in high school and college, they should be their own best advocates. Below are a number of considerations when advocating for your child.

• Understand how your child processes information and how she or he learns best. Consider the way in which communication occurs in the classroom. Some children, especially those with ADHD, predominantly the inattentive type, or those with language disorders, process information more slowly. Consequently, when several directions are given at one time (e.g., "Get out your homework paper, your study guide, and your book"), the child with ADHD may still be looking for the first item when it is time for the child to respond to a question from the teacher. In contrast, some children with ADHD, predominantly the hyperactive/impulsive type, need information presented in an upbeat, fast rate of speed before they become bored.

- Children with ADHD present fewer behavior problems when there are routines and schedules within the classroom. If your child is placed in an environment in which she or he knows what is expected throughout the day, there will be fewer off-task behaviors. More disruptive behavior occurs during unstructured time (e.g., passing of papers to the neighbor, trips down the hall).

- Children with attentional problems tend to be more attentive and experience fewer behavior outbursts when they are in a classroom where the teacher moves around and remains in close proximity to the students. Teachers who remain at their desk will typically not provide the best setting for children with ADHD. Some children may function best if they are seated in the middle-front section of the classroom rather than on the side front or in the back of the room. The location of the child's desk will depend on a number of variables (e.g., the activity of the classroom, teacher location, distractions). For example, most teachers report that they usually place the child with ADHD near the teacher's desk. This may be fine in some classrooms; however, many times this is the busiest location in the classroom. This location may be too distracting for the child with ADHD. If you think your child's location in the room is a problem, you may request that an objective observer evaluate to determine the best location for your child.

- Consider the way in which the classroom is organized. When completing independent work, children seated at individual desks rather than at tables have been shown to produce more work. This will reduce talking and disruptive behavior. A table-setting format (i.e., desks pushed together to form a rectangle) promotes socialization, whereas rows of desks promote on-task behavior. Classrooms with four walls and a door reduce the noise and activity level. Open classrooms can result in more aggressive and disruptive behaviors.

- Children with ADHD demonstrate more appropriate behavior when the teacher posts the rules for the classroom and each student is aware of the mild consequence for each rule violation. When a consequence is given, the child with disruptive behaviors does better when the reason is clearly stated. For example, "Matthew, your feet were not under your desk; you kicked Jeffrey; put your name in my discipline book." Rules can be more easily followed and recalled when the following guidelines are used:

1. There should be a limited number of rules, no more than four to six.

2. The rules should be specific and simple. For example, "Be responsible" is too vague. A rule such as "Homework should be returned the day it is due" is specific and clear.

3. Rules that are phrased in the positive are better. By phrasing the rule in the positive, it is clearer what the child should do rather than what she or he should *not* do. Rather than stating a rule such as "No interrupting when the teacher is talking," state it as "Raise your hand and be recognized before speaking in class."

4. Rules are better if they can be observed and counted. For example, a rule such as "Pay attention" cannot be counted; however, a rule such as "Keep your eyes on the teacher when she is talking" can be observed and counted.

5. Your child should be able to tell you the rules of the classroom and what the consequence is for a specific rule violation. If your child is unable to tell you

the rules of the classroom, ask the teacher and then discuss these rules with your child at home. You cannot expect your child to follow the rules if she or he does not know what they are. If mild consequences are given immediately following a rule violation, the child will be better able to understand and follow the rules. The rules do not need to be different for the child with ADHD if these guidelines are followed.

6. The rules are more effective if they are posted. For the child with ADHD, it is helpful for teachers or parents to discuss with the children the rules during the first week of school and review them each Monday and after a holiday.

- Teachers who use the overhead projector rather than the chalkboard for instruction have a better view of the children. The teacher can then determine whether the children understand what is being presented. If a child is absent one day, the child can copy the material that was presented on the day she or he was absent if the overheads are saved.

Additional interventions that may be considered by the support team include strategies and activities that provide for a more *interactive learning environment*. When children who have ADHD are in classrooms that permit the students to interact more with their teachers, they appear to do better. Consider the following when determining reasons for your child's difficulties:

- Children with ADHD do better in classrooms where more discussions are conducted. The teacher could allow for this by occasionally asking a child to clarify a point or to ask a child a question related to the topic of discussion. By allowing a child to repeat a comment made by another child, better listening and attending skills are promoted. If a teacher habitually repeats what a child contributed to the discussion, children are being trained that they do not need to listen to the contributions of other children.

- Teachers who use effective questioning techniques promote better listening skills. When the teacher only lectures, the children will begin to tune the teacher out. The teacher can include the children in the lesson by occasionally asking individual children to answer questions or to ask for unison responses.

- Students are engaged more in their learning when teachers provide for more hands-on activities.

- Teachers who change activities often, moving from passive activities to active ones, maintain better attention from their students.

Since most students with ADHD experience difficulty with organizational skills, your child will likely need some assistance in this area. Specific strategies that may help your child include the following:

- Require your child to have a backpack for books and other school materials. Regularly require your child to clean out the backpack. You may initially need to assist your child with this project.

- Require your child to use a three-ring notebook with several two-sided pockets and a pencil pouch. This will be needed more when your child reaches the third grade or when homework assignments are given. The child should have a designated place for assignments that need to be completed and assignments to turn in the next day.

- Insist that your child use a monthly assignment calendar. If you start this practice early, it will be a habit by the time your child reaches high school. You may want the support team to consider having the teacher or the child's peer partner check to determine whether the assignments are correctly entered. The teacher or peer/buddy should initial the assignment if it is written correctly, and then you should initial it after the assignment has been completed. If there is no homework assignment, this should be written and initialed also. This will prevent your child from telling you that there is no homework simply because she or he forgot to write it in the book. You can add this to the point system you have already begun.

• If your child experiences difficulty getting home with handouts, ask the teacher if your child could have the handouts with the holes already punched so that they can be placed in the notebook immediately. Many children with organizational problems lose their handouts before they get home because they stuff them in books or book bags. This practice of having the holes already punched will help to eliminate this problem.

• Ask for instruction in study skills when your child reaches middle school. *Skills for School Success*, by Anita Archer and Mary Gleason (Curriculum Associates, 1989), is an excellent study skills workbook. *Study Strategies Made Easy: A Practical Plan for School Success* (Specialty Press, 1996), by Leslie Davis, Sandi Sirotowitz, and Harvey Parker, is a practical book that teaches students in Grades 6 through 12 how to learn. This can be purchased through the A.D.D. WareHouse. Don't assume that just because your child has reached middle school, she or he will know how to take notes. Most children, and especially those with ADHD or a learning disability, will need specific instruction in note taking.

• It is likely that most students with ADHD will need homework monitoring to some degree for some time. Any changes in this monitoring will need to be gradual. Don't be embarrassed to ask for this assistance from the teachers.

Other accommodations that may be considered by the support team for the child with ADHD or a learning disability are suggested below.

• Your child's learning may be better facilitated when the teacher uses a multisensory approach to learning new material. For example, when studying the human heart, the children could touch and feel a pig's heart in addition to talking about it.

• When the child with ADHD is allowed to move around after being required to sit for a long time period, attention and concentration are improved.

• Ask your child's teachers if the word processor can be used to complete long written assignments.

• Ask your child's support team if your child can be permitted to select another way to present the information learned. For example, one time during the month, each child can select one assignment to present in a different format—an oral presentation of a book report rather than a written one, a poster describing the events in a story rather than a written report, and so on.

• If your child has weaknesses in peer relationships, suggest that the school consider adopting a social skills curriculum. The entire school could have a social skill for the week. Each teacher would teach the skill to children in his or her class at the beginning of the week, and all school staff (e.g., cafeteria workers, principals, teachers, volunteers) would reinforce any child they observe using the social skill appropriately. This helps with generalization. As problem behaviors arise within the school, new social skills could be added.

▶ Step 2: If your child continues to struggle despite the implementation of interventions and modifications in the regular classroom, the support team may recommend a comprehensive evaluation to determine if your child is eligible for special education services.

Under IDEA (Part B of the Individuals with Disabilities Education Act), the school will evaluate a child who is suspected of having a disability. This evaluation is completed by professionals in the school system at no charge to the family.

▶ Step 3: If a child is diagnosed with ADHD, a learning disability, or another disability, a team of professionals and the parent(s) meet to discuss the child's eligibility for special education services (called variously the IEP team meeting, M-Team, or Multidisciplinary Team).

A child with ADHD can qualify for special education services under the category of "Other Health Impaired" (in some states this is referred to as "Health Impaired"), a learning disability, or a serious emotional disability if the diagnostic criteria is met for the disability. Your child would only need to meet the criteria for one of these disabilities to be considered eligible for special education services.

▶ Step 4: If this team of professionals and the child's parents determine that your child is eligible for special education services through one of the recognized disabilities in the federal IDEA guidelines, the team will develop an Individualized Education Plan (IEP) to address your child's deficit areas, which can include academic, behavior, social functioning, and/or adaptive functioning.

▶ Step 5: Once the child is found eligible for special education services, the team will meet at least one time during each school year to write and/or modify your child's IEP.

The team can meet more frequently if the parents or school personnel believe the child's program is not appropriately meeting her or his needs. These meetings will continue throughout the child's years in school or until the child is no longer eligible for special education services. In order to determine that a child is no longer eligible for special education services, the school must reevaluate the child, and the child must no longer meet the certification criteria for a disability as outlined under the IDEA guidelines.

▶ Step 6: This team of professionals is also responsible for writing a transition plan for your child.

If your child is provided services under IDEA, the school must develop a plan that will assist the student when making the transition from the school environment to the post-secondary environment (e.g., college, career, social relationships). It is recommended that the foundations for transition planning begin when the student is in the elementary or middle school grades; however, the plan must begin no later than 14 years of age (Halpern, 1994). Most schools will attach an Individual Transition Plan (ITP) to the IEP. Wehman (1995) has developed a guide that is useful in developing these plans. This guide can be obtained through PRO-ED in Austin, Texas. The guide is titled *Individual Transition Plans: The Teacher's Curriculum Guide for Helping Youth with Special Needs*. If your child's team has not begun to develop a transition plan when your teen reaches 14 years of age, ask about this at your annual meeting.

? *What is your role as a parent in the education of your child?*

In addition to being an advocate for your child and teaching your child to be her or his own advocate, you are also equal partners with school professionals in educating your child. Although you should not be required to teach the subject material to your child, you do have certain responsibilities in supporting the education of your child. Several parents have found it helpful to observe in the child's classroom one full day at the beginning of the school year. By doing this, the parent can support the child in learning the routines in the classroom (e.g., location for turning in assignments, behavior rules for the classroom and hallway). This observation would not be appropriate for most children in middle or high school. These students are likely to be embarrassed when a parent observes in the classroom.

Another role of the parent is to establish a study plan for or with your child. This should be done prior to the start of the school year and should be maintained throughout the year. A homework routine should definitely be established for the student in middle or high school. One of the most frequent behaviors that result in poor performance in school is the failure to complete homework. While modifications may be needed due to changes in the student's activities, the routine should not be eliminated. The following homework routine has been adapted from the work of Forgatch and Patterson (1989):

1. *First, decide how much time your child should study each day.* To determine how much is an appropriate amount of time, consult with the classroom teacher. Many schools recommend that homework assignments take approximately 15 minutes for each grade/year in school. For example, a first-grade student should spend no more than 15 minutes each evening completing homework, a second-grader 30 minutes, and a third grader 45 minutes. It is rare, however, that homework time should extend beyond 1 hour for the elementary-aged child. It has been noted that it typically takes a child with ADHD or a learning disability three times as long to complete an assignment at home as it would during the school day. Thus, if an assignment at school is not completed, and it is sent home to be completed, the time to complete it would be tripled. A 10-minute assignment would usually take 30 minutes to complete at home. This practice of sending schoolwork home to be completed should be avoided. If this is occurring, schedule a meeting with your child's teacher to develop another plan. In addition, if your elementary-aged child is spending hours completing homework, discuss this with the teacher. Your child also needs a life outside of school.

2. *Select a regular time in which homework should be completed.* Try to keep this consistent 5 days per week (Sunday through Thursday or Monday through Friday). Even if your child reports that there is no homework, require the study time to remain as scheduled. The child could read a book, write a letter, write in a daily journal, or work on some other enrichment project. Immediately after school, most children need a brief break and a snack before beginning homework assignments. Usually, immediately after the snack and break is a good time to complete homework assignments. If children wait until after they have eaten dinner, they are usually too tired. On the other hand, some parents have found that homework can be completed more quickly and with greater accuracy if the time is scheduled while the effects of medication are still in the child's system. You and your child need to decide the best time for completion of homework.

3. *During this regularly scheduled time, the house should be relatively quiet.* Everyone should be doing something constructive (e.g., reading the newspaper, reading a book, cooking dinner). Do not allow other children to watch television while the child with ADHD is completing her or his homework assignments. This will be too distracting. Some children may attend better if there is "white noise" or instrumental music playing. You will need to assess this by determining the amount of work completed under these conditions. It is rare, however, for a child to attend better with a visual distraction, such as the television.

4. *Select the location for homework completion.* The child should have a desk with good lighting. If the child does not have a desk or table in her or his room, arrange an environment in another part of the house that is established as the work area.

5. *Provide the necessary supplies for homework completion.* This may include paper, crayons, scissors, tape, pencils, erasers, notebooks, and book bags. For the young child, an activity that involves purchasing these supplies with a parent helps set the stage for its importance. Many parents report that they purchase another set of books to use at home. If the school will allow you to obtain another set of books, this will reduce some of your headaches. This is a well-accepted practice across the country, so do not hesitate to ask for this accommodation if you think it will help.

6. *Check occasionally to see if your child is working.* Use this time to be an encourager, not a snoop to point out what is being done wrong. Look for something your child is doing right, rather than nagging about inappropriate behavior. Some children will need more help than others with their work. If your child needs help, show him or her how to do the first problem, do the second problem with her or him, and have your child do one by himself or herself. This is the "I do, we do, you do" approach as presented in an earlier chapter. It works well with children with learning problems. Then establish a reinforcement system that will provide your child with support and structure. For example, set the portable timer for 10 minutes and state, "I will do one problem for every 5 you accurately complete in the next 10 minutes." You can gradually increase the number of problems you expect your child to complete in this time period.

7. *Build in some incentives for following the study schedule.* We know that children with learning disabilities or ADHD need a more supportive environment than those without these disabilities. Other children may be motivated by the internal satisfaction that is derived when a task is completed. Children with ADHD often need external motivators. As they get older, it is hoped that these children will also be internally motivated; however, most do not have this motivation during childhood or early adolescence. For example, an incentive plan that permits the child to earn 30 minutes of television time, telephone time, or outside play for each assignment completed may be helpful. Another consideration would be to include this on your point system, as Heather's parents did in Figure 6.4.

8. *Take an interest in your child's experiences at school.* Be compassionate and listen to what is being communicated; however, you do not have to find solutions to all the problems. Comment on what is done right in school, rather then pointing out the negatives. Encourage your child, but let her or him know that you also support the school. If your child hears you speak negatively about the school, she or he will likely adopt that thinking as well. Many parents want their children to share their school experiences the minute they walk through the door. This approach is annoying to many children, especially adolescents. Avoid quizzing your child the minute the door opens. Wait until your child is ready to share information with you.

? What should you do when the homework routine is not enough and your child continues to do poorly?

Even with a consistently followed homework routine, there are times when a child may struggle. Common problems presented by children with ADHD include a failure to turn in homework assignments even when they are completed, behavior problems at school, and failure to complete school assignments. The best approach to dealing with these persistent problems is for the school and the home to collaborate to find a potential solution. If a 504 plan or an IEP has been written, these solutions could be written into the child's plan. The following procedure is recommended when your child continues to experience school-related problems even after you have implemented a homework routine:

1. *Contact your child's teacher to schedule a meeting to discuss your concerns.* At this meeting, avoid setting the stage for an adversarial relationship. Most of the time, if concerns are expressed appropriately, the teacher will respond positively. If, however, you go into the meeting blaming the teacher, the teacher will likely become defensive, and relatively little will be accomplished. Express your concern about your child's performance and let the teacher know what you have tried to date (e.g., homework routine). Then ask for the teacher's help. Use your good listening techniques for this conference and avoid making assumptions about the teacher's behavior.

Good communication skills include using the feedback technique that utilizes more "I messages" than "you messages." For example, "I am concerned about Harrison's incomplete assignments. Can we identify a plan that may help him to complete these at school?" works better than making a statement such as, "Why do *you* send all Harrison's school assignments to do at home? Can't *you* get him to do them at school?" Giving "you messages" typically results in defensiveness on the part of the teacher. This is also a good time to use the STPDE plan for problem solving, as described in Chapter 7. Remain on task and stick to the problem to be solved, rather than attacking the teacher.

2. *Work with the teacher to establish a way to monitor your child's school performance or behavior.* Most teachers will respond positively to this approach if it does not require excessive time on their part. Before developing a plan, both the teacher and parent should determine two or three behaviors that need improvement. Avoid listing too many behaviors at first. Start small, with two or three problem behaviors that you and the teacher have identified. Remember that these must be observable and countable. Select one behavior that is disruptive to the classroom and one or two academic problems (or vice versa depending on the primary problems of the child). Possible behaviors to consider include turning in homework assignments, raising hand before talking, and having paper and pencil ready when class begins. If possible, these behaviors should be expressed in the positive ("start behaviors" rather than "stop behaviors").

The key is to select the behaviors for which both you and the teacher can easily see progress and set the goal at such a level that the child is able to be successful during the first week. Rather than focusing on grades and only rewarding good grades, focus on the behaviors that can result in good grades. In other words, *reward the effort, rather than only the product.* Remember, it often takes more effort for the child with ADHD than it does other children. See Figure 8.1 for an example of a School Monitoring Card, a method to obtain daily feedback from the teacher.

3. *Either the teacher or the parent should share the School Monitoring Card with the child.* At this time, you and your child can select reinforcers to be included in the menu of rewards and the number of points (or +'s) that are needed to obtain these rewards (see Figure 6.3). You may add bonus points for bringing home the point chart each day. If you are already using a point chart at home, add these behaviors to this one rather than making a new one (see Figure 6.4). Keep the point chart simple. If you make it too difficult to monitor, you will not follow through.

4. *Gradually increase the standards for which your child can earn points.* As progress is made, new behaviors can be added to the chart and old ones can be deleted. The key to success, however, is to make changes gradually. Don't abruptly stop the program. You may need to change your rewards to maintain a high level of motivation. School suspension should be avoided if at all possible. If your child is suspended more than twice during the school year, ask your child's teachers to convene an M-Team if your child is in special education, or request a 504 meeting if your child is not in special education. If your child is being suspended, this is an indication that the academic placement is not meeting her or his needs; thus, changes or modifications may be needed.

Josh's School Monitoring Card

Date:_____

Behavior	7:30–9:00	9:00–10:30	10:30–12:30	12:30–2:30
1. Keeps hands and feet in place.	+	+	+	+
2. Waits for directions to be given before beginning work.	+	–	–	+
3. Completes classroom assignment.	–	+	–	+

Parent's Signature	Child's Signature	Teacher's Signature

FIGURE 8.1. Sample School Monitoring Card.

? My child seems too old to use a School Monitoring Card; what else can I do?

As your child gets older (fourth or fifth grade through high school), it is often beneficial to involve the student in developing a contract. This procedure tends to work best when the school selects one teacher or another professional in the school to be your child's coach or case manager. This person should have a positive relationship with your child, be able to meet with your child on a regular basis (at least at the beginning of each week and at the end of each week), be able to communicate well with teachers and parents, and have the ability to help your child set priorities for the week. Below are the procedures for implementing a weekly goal contract (adapted from the work of William Pelham, 1995).

1. *Determine the goals that are appropriate for the student.* The case manager or coach will discuss the child's needs with teachers and other school personnel. The older child or adolescent should also be involved in the selection of these goals. Select two to three behavioral or academic goals that can be measured on a daily basis. Keep these goals until the child has reached mastery. New goals can be selected to replace these as needs change.

2. *Specifically define each goal.* Specifically and clearly define each goal, and phrase it in the positive if at all possible. For example, try "George will wait to begin work until directions have been given" rather than "Do not begin work until directions are given." For this goal to be effective, the child should know specifically what "to wait" means. Does this mean that the child will pause for 3 seconds before beginning the assignment?

3. *Determine how severe the problem is, and set the criterion for each goal.* One way to do this is to count the number of times the behavior occurs or does not occur for 3 days. For example, if you want the student to reduce the number of times she or he interrupts the teacher (or talks back to the teacher), determine how many times this behavior is occurring. If she or he interrupts an average of 120 times per day, a goal of fewer than 100 interruptions per day may be appropriate for the first week's goal. In contrast, if the student interrupts 30 times per day, the goal of fewer than 24 interruptions per day would be appropriate. Usually, reducing the goal by 20% each week is attainable for most students. The first week that the Weekly Goal Contract is used, set the criterion at a level at which you know the student will be able to reach each goal. If you set the

goals too high, the student will feel defeated before he or she even starts. For example, prior to using the Weekly Contract, Harrison returned his homework 45% of the time; thus, a goal of 50% was an improvement, but it was not too difficult.

4. *The coach should explain the Goal Sheet to the student.* If the parent is unaware of the goals that have been selected, inform the parent also. The coach (case manager) should meet briefly with the student at the beginning of each week to discuss the goals for the week. (See Figure 8.2 for a sample goal plan and Appendix C for a blank Weekly Goal Contract form.) The older the individual, the more involved she or he should be in the process of goal selection as well as in setting the criterion for attainment of each goal. For example, the middle school student may select one goal, and the school staff could select the other goals.

5. *The parents and student should select the rewards to be given at home if the goals are reached.* At the end of each week, the student should take home the results of the contract. Parents will provide the prearranged rewards for the goals that have been reached. If assistance is needed in selecting appropriate rewards, the parent should discuss these with the coach or review the reward guidelines in this book. It is critical that this home-based reward system be implemented consistently and that the rewards are motivating to the child. This reinforcement system is more likely to change behaviors when the parents, rather than the school, provide the reward or when rewards are provided in both locations.

6. *Modify the program as needed.* At the end of the week, when the Goal Sheet was reviewed with Harrison, the criterion for each goal was gradually raised because he had reached mastery of the current goals. Changes in the goals should always be made

---

Weekly Goal Contract

This week's goals are the following:

1. Harrison will turn in at least 50% of his homework each day of the week.

2. Harrison agrees to be on time for 50% of his classes during the week (on time for 15 of the 30 classes for the week).

3. Harrison agrees to bring the necessary materials and supplies to his English and math classes each day of the week (e.g., pencils, books, paper).

If **Harrison**
Student's Name
reaches the goals,

he will be allowed to park in the principal's parking space for one week and drive the family car to school for one week.
Reward

If **Harrison**
Student's Name
does *not* reach the goals,

he will wash the family car on the weekend, and he will ride the school bus to school the following week.
Consequence

| Student's Signature | Date | Coach's Signature | Date |

| Parent's Signature | Date | Parent's Signature | Date |

FIGURE 8.2. Sample Weekly Goal Contract.

gradually. If the program is stopped suddenly, the student will likely revert back to the original behaviors. In addition, if the program drags on too long without modifications, the child will likely lose motivation and regress. The key is to make all changes gradually. By gradually increasing the criterion to reach each goal and by changing the rewards occasionally, good improvement can occur. The coach should meet briefly with the student at the beginning of the week to remind the student of the goals and to discuss any obstacles that might interfere with goal attainment.

7. *If the program is not working to improve the child's behavior, ask the following questions:*

- Are the goals appropriate for this person?

- Are the criteria realistic?

- Do the school staff, child, and parent have a clear understanding of the definition of each goal?

- Is everyone consistently following through with her or his role in the contract (e.g., Is the coach meeting with the student at least at the beginning of the week and at the end of the week to discuss progress and plans? Is the coach someone the student likes? Are teachers recording appropriate behaviors? Are parents and school personnel consistently providing the reward? Are the rewards powerful enough to change the behavior?)

- Is the student taking home the Goal Sheet at the end of the week?

- Is the student receiving more positive feedback than negative consequences during any given day? If not, changes need to occur in the contract.

Final Notes

As you can easily recognize, the job of parenting and educating a child with ADHD is not easy. It may seem overwhelming at times, but this chapter has presented a number of suggestions that you and the school personnel can implement and that can result in positive changes in your child. As you can readily recognize, medication is not the only treatment that can be used when educating a child with ADHD. Below are some of the key points to remember from this chapter.

- Be a good advocate for your child. Present your concerns in a caring and positive manner that will result in positive changes for your child.

- Know what to expect in 504 meetings, IEP meetings, and Transition Planning meetings. The more informed you are, the more productive these meetings can be.

- Know your child. Where are your child's strengths and weaknesses? Suggest ideas to the school that will address your child's weak areas and will allow your child to use her or his strengths. Your child must experience some success during the school day.

- Establish a homework routine for (or with) your child.

- Collaborate with your child's teachers and implement the Daily School Monitoring Card or the Weekly Goal Plan if needed.

- Communicate regularly with your child's teacher. This does not mean that you should be at the school every day, but you should meet more than once each year. If you have a daily or weekly goal plan, your communication can be through this format.

Questions Asked by Parents of Children with ADHD

I t is impossible to cover all the problems and issues concerning parents of children with ADHD in one book. This chapter contains questions that have been asked by parents of children with ADHD. These are real questions asked by parents who have participated in Vanderbilt's Summer Day Treatment Program. Frequently there is no one answer that can solve a problem. Each family is different and each circumstance may be different. Thus, these answers are only *possible solutions*. If the problem persists, even after carefully following the principles detailed in this book, consult a professional with experience and training in working with children and adolescents with disruptive behaviors.

? *When I go to the grocery store or to a department store to shop, my 6-year-old manages to get into trouble. It never fails. I can't get a babysitter each time I have to go to the store. What can I do to make this a better experience?*

When your child has become adept at responding to your commands at home, he or she is more likely to follow your requests while in public. One important guideline for managing behavior in public is to *establish the rules before you leave the house*. Make the rules brief and few (two or three). For example, for a young child the rules might be (1) stand close to me at all times; (2) ask permission before touching something; (3) do not beg (if you ask for something, use an appropriate voice). For older children, rules are still needed, but they may not be as restrictive.

Next, *establish a behavior plan for following your rules*. One approach is to inform your child that you will be observing for positive behaviors or when rules have been followed. When you observe your child following a rule, provide immediate positive feedback. If your child also needs a tangible reward, you may decide to give one chip. Your child can cash these chips in for special privileges when she or he arrives home (e.g., for each chip earned, your child earns 5 minutes of computer time).

Another approach, however somewhat less desirable, is to give your child 10 chips or 10 points before entering the public place. For each rule violation, the child loses one chip or point. The remaining chips can be cashed in at the end of the trip or added to the point/chip system at home. For example, each chip could be equivalent to one dime; thus, at the end of the trip your child could use the money to purchase something or save it for the chip system used at home. One parent of a six-year-old boy has used the following procedure with success:

▶ Each time a rule was violated, his mother calmly informed him of the rule violation ("Michael, you did not ask permission before touching the bread. You punched a hole in the bread.") and put a mark on the child's hand with an ink pen. The consequence was that he had to spend 1 minute in time-out for each mark made on his hand. He was not allowed to wash his hand until he had served his time-out. If he had no marks on his hand at the end of the trip, he was permitted to stop at the ice cream store on the way home.

Finally, *have a clear set of consequences for misbehavior or noncompliance.* Remember that mild forms of punishment are more effective than severe forms of punishment. Failure to earn chips/points may be a sufficient consequence for some children. In review, it is critical that you reinforce your child for appropriate behavior and not take the positive behavior for granted and be sure to remind your child of the rules before entering the public place. Another word of caution: If you know your child is tired and hungry, avoid public places at that time.

? *I am going on a vacation with my family. How can the trip be pleasant with my child who has ADHD? He hates traveling in the car, and he is always picking on his sister.*

Again, as in the previous example, establish the rules, reinforcers, and consequences prior to taking the trip. Make sure your rules are appropriate and are ones that you can easily enforce. Also, plan ahead. If your children are young, plan appropriate car activities (e.g., bring materials for drawing, books to look at, listen to, or read).

▶ One parent was taking her children to Florida for a vacation. She determined that she usually gave her children approximately $15 to spend in any way they might choose when they had reached their destination. She gave each child $15 in quarters (all children, not just the child with ADHD). Before the trip, she explained the rules to the children, "Each time either of you breaks a rule (picking at sister, yelling, etc.), you must give me one quarter." This approach worked great for this parent. The children's behavior was improved from previous trips, and each child arrived in Florida with approximately $13. The key is to plan ahead; don't just hope for the best. She had also planned several activities for the children while in the car (books on tape, crossword puzzles, crayons, paper).

Another set of parents used the above procedure traveling to their destination, but they were worried that the return trip would be disastrous. He and his wife decided to use the following procedure:

▶ On the return trip, he and his wife obtained several rolls of dimes. The children were told that they would prepare each child a sandwich and water for the return trip. In order to earn money to buy additional food items (e.g., soft drinks, potato chips, candy) for their trip home, the children were required to demonstrate positive behaviors. Thus, when a positive behavior or comment was demonstrated, a parent provided the child with positive feedback and one dime. During the family's periodic stops, each child could purchase the additional food items she or he wanted. The children were so busy thinking of positive ways to interact that there were relatively few negative behaviors.

Both of these parents demonstrated a sense of humor that has helped them in their interactions with their children. They have been willing to attempt new approaches to their parenting and have enjoyed the challenges of the job. One of the biggest obstacles that many parents must overcome in their parenting of children with ADHD is their rigidity in their parenting style. Parenting a child with ADHD requires a great deal of creative thinking and the ability to predict situations that may be problematic and then plan for them.

? *How do I get my child to stop arguing with me?*

One approach that may work involves the use of a cassette recorder. William Jenson, from the University of Utah, recommends placing a cassette recorder in front of your child when she or he begins arguing and saying to the child, "Argue into this if you want to argue. I'm not going to argue with you." This will usually stop the arguing. Remember that it takes two people to have an argument. If your child is arguing with you about a rule that is nonnegotiable, stand firm, provide your teen with the reasons for your decision, but do not argue. One mother of a teen son who was ADHD had the following discussion when he asked his mother if he could go to a co-ed sleepover. This was one of her nonnegotiable rules.

GREG: Why can't I go to the sleepover? All my other friends are going.

MOTHER: Greg, this is not negotiable. Your dad and I have agreed that this is not appropriate for 15-year-olds. It opens the door for pressures that you are not ready to handle.

GREG: Mom, I'm just tired of it! You're always getting your morals from God. Can't you ever think for yourself?

This situation easily could have evolved into an argument; however, Greg's mother explained her reasons for the decision and that it was not negotiable. If Greg knows there are other situations in which the decision is negotiable, he will be more likely to accept his mother's answer to this request. The older children are, the more involved they can be in the decision making about those rules that are negotiable.

If you find that you have gotten yourself into an argument with your child, tell the child or teen that you need a break and that you will resume the conversation when you have calmed down. After you both have had sufficient time to regain control of your emotions, resume your conversation and begin by apologizing. Next, ask your child or teen for her or his opinion on the situation. This will let your child know that you want to hear her or his opinion and will weigh your child's viewpoint when making the final decision. It may not change the final decision, but your child will feel that her or his opinion has merit.

When children are between the ages of 7 and 10 years, it is normal for them to respond as if they were defending their statement or position. They often want to get in the last word. At this age, a sense of fairness is being developed. Sometimes the "last word" may really be an explanation of why something was done a certain way, rather than an argument. For example, Travis was scolded by his father for leaving his shoes on the front porch where the dog could take them off. Travis responded, "Mom told me to leave them there until I cleaned the mud off the bottoms." This response was likely an explanation because he felt that the scolding was not fair. If Dad responds with another reprimand, an argument might ensue. Carefully listen to your child's comments before automatically interpreting them as "talking back."

When trying to determine why your child appears to be arguing a great deal, first evaluate your family's mode of communication. Do you and your spouse argue a great deal? Some parents are not aware of this until they have heard their child's responses. If this is the case, you may discuss with your child the difference between "talking back" and discussing a topic and to remain aware of the tone you set when you are having a discussion.

▶ The parents of one 10-year-old had determined that their child's "talking back" and arguing were occurring far too frequently. They did not object to

Jason's talking to them about differences of opinion, but his tone of voice was most offensive. First, they discussed with their son the issues related to "talking back." They presented several role-plays and discussed appropriate and inappropriate ways to express feelings. Since they were already using a point chart with their son, they were able to easily add this to the point system. They included the following behaviors: (1) "Jason will have an argument-free morning prior to going to school." (2) "Jason will have an argument-free afternoon before dinner." (3) "Jason will have an argument-free evening." He was permitted to discuss issues with his parents, but an appropriate tone of voice was required. For each behavior for which the criterion was met, he was awarded 10 points. This approach worked for some time, and then the behaviors were gradually faded from the point system. During the following year, the number of arguments increased again. The parents and Jason discussed the issue again, and it was decided that Jason would lose points each time he argued using a sarcastic tone of voice.

As is the case with many of our children, you may have to revisit a behavior occasionally and establish a new approach to working with a child with a problem behavior.

? *My child "invents" facts and situations. It has almost become automatic for me to ask, "Is that true?" It's usually an elaboration of something that happened. I try to matter-of-factly emphasize the truth about the thing he is describing and tell him that he has a great imagination, but this is pretty frustrating and scary. He is 9 years old. I teach him about the importance of telling the truth and encourage him to do so. I hesitate to just punish him for lying. . . . Help!*

It is important to recognize that there are different reasons for lying. Children who are of preschool age cannot readily distinguish between fact and fantasy. This is not lying by definition. A lie is an untrue statement with the intent to deceive. A preschooler does not intend to deceive you by saying that he talked to Santa last night. Most children do not begin to distinguish a truth from a falsehood until they are about 6 years of age. I recall my own son, as a 6-year-old, telling the neighbor a falsehood when asked if he had any brothers and sisters. He said, "Well I have two sisters (a true statement), and I have five brothers, but Mom makes them live in the attic (a false statement)." When questioned by the neighbor about the five brothers who lived in the attic, he later recounted, "Oh, they aren't real brothers, they're spiders." At 6, Thomas was able to distinguish between a falsehood and the truth although he was still experimenting in some fantasy.

Schaefer and Millman (1981) discussed Piaget's theory that children go through three phases of lying. In phase 1, the child believes that a lie is wrong because a punishment follows the lying. If the parent does not punish the child for lying then it must mean that it's okay to lie. In phase 2 of lying, the child believes that lying is wrong, and even if the child is not punished, she or he still knows it is wrong. In phase 3, the individual knows that lying is wrong out of respect for the other person. Some believe that only about one third of children reach this third phase by age 12 years. Chess and Thomas (1987) presented Kohlberg's theory of moral development in his study of adolescent males. Kohlberg defined six stages of moral judgment and ranked them in order from the most immature to the most mature level. In the earliest stage, "rules are followed when they are in the immediate interest of the child," and in the next stage, "goodness is equated with helping and pleasing others." In the most mature stage (sixth stage), "moral judgments are based on self-accepted universal principles of justice." Kohlberg's work suggests that only a small minority of adults reach the highest stage of moral development (Chess & Thomas, 1987, p. 186).

Each of us has probably lied at some time in our lives. Thomas Phelan, in his book, *1-2-3: Magic!*, states that children lie primarily for two reasons: (1) to impress others or (2) to get out of trouble ("Watergate lying"). Schaefer and Millman (1981) describe 10 reasons for children to lie. These include the following:

1. Self-defense: To escape the unpleasant consequences of a behavior, such as parental disapproval or punishment.

2. Denial: A way of handling painful memories, feelings, or fantasies.

3. Modeling: Copying the behavior of adults.

4. Ego-boasting: Boasting to receive attention or admiration.

5. Reality-testing: Attempting to find out the difference between reality and fantasy.

6. Loyalty: Protection of other children.

7. Hostility: Act of general hostility toward others.

8. Gain: To get something for oneself.

9. Self-image: The child has been told repeatedly that she is a liar and has come to believe it.

10. Distrust: Parents tend not to trust and believe a child when he tells the truth, so the child prefers to lie. (pp. 310–311)

Most children with ADHD or other disruptive behavior disorders lie to get out of trouble. They want to avoid the punishment or the yelling that often follows a misbehavior, and they find that lying about it is easier than facing the consequence (Phelan, 1984). While lying is not that uncommon for young children, it is a behavior that needs to be targeted for extinction if it becomes a consistent pattern after the child reaches 6 years of age.

As suggested earlier in this book, it is easier to prevent a negative behavior from occurring than to stop one after it has become a habit for the child. First, evaluate your behavior to determine whether you may be contributing to your child's problem with lying. Phelan reports that one reason a child may lie is that the parents have trained the child to lie. To determine whether you are training your child to lie, ask yourself the following questions:

• Do you become overly upset when your child does something wrong? Do you yell, scream, or spank your child when she or he does something wrong? If you do, you may be giving your child a motive to lie. Your child rationalizes that he or she might be able to avoid the punishment by lying, so the child will take her or his chances in hopes that she or he won't get caught.

• When your child was in the earliest stage of lying, did your child receive a consequence for lying, or did you think it was cute?

Another way to reinforce lying is to interrogate your child in an attempt to find out what really happened. Your child may respond in order to cover it up. It might go like this:

FATHER: Where did you get the money to buy those toys?

BEN:	I found it.
FATHER:	Where did you find it?
BEN:	I forgot.
FATHER:	You've got to know where you found it if you found it. Now, where did it come from?
BEN:	Oh yeah, I forgot, my teacher gave it to me for helping her.
FATHER:	Listen young man, are you lying to me? Your mother is missing $10 from her billfold, and she caught you in her purse.
BEN:	I didn't steal it; Matt did, and he gave it to me.

What was happening in this situation? Why did the child continue to lie? The child's father was backing him into a corner; he didn't want to get into trouble; the child got nervous; he lied to avoid the consequence.

How can a parent extinguish this type of lying?

- *Apply the minimal talking and no-emotion rules.* In other words, remain as calm as possible and do not lecture. The more upset you become, the greater the child's motive for lying.

- *Do not interrogate your child.* If you already know that your child did it, simply inform her or him of this and administer the punishment. Do not provide your child with the opportunity to lie by asking what happened. If you do not know what happened, then accept the answer as truth and keep your comments brief. If you find out later that your child lied, inform her or him of what you found out, punish for the original offense, and then punish for the lying (Phelan, 1984, p. 44).

Other techniques that help to promote honesty include the following:

- Model honesty. If you make a practice of telling "white lies," your child may mimic your behavior.

- Discuss moral questions related to lies and honesty. Remember the level of moral development of your child. Don't expect her or him to avoid lying because it the right thing to do when she or he is only 5 years of age. You may read several books on this topic and discuss them with your child. An appropriate book for children who are between 4 and 8 years of age is *Sam, Bangs, and Moonshine*, by E. M. Ness (Holt, Rinehart & Winston, 1966). For the older child (ages 10–13), try *The Bad Times of Irma Bawnlein*, by C. R. Brink (Simon & Schuster, 1972). Your local library or bookstore may have other books appropriate for family discussion.

Some children who develop a pattern of lying behavior may also exhibit stealing behavior. Patterson (1975) reports that by the age of 5 or 6, most children have learned to stop stealing and fewer than 1 child in 10 continues to steal at a high rate. Patterson also suggests that if a child has a problem with aggressive behavior, she or he has a 50-50 chance of also having a problem with stealing. Patterson suggests that if a child continues to steal more than once a month at 5 or 6 years of age, you should consider this a problem behavior that needs intervention. Even if your child is stealing small items at a high rate, it will likely become a bigger problem if it is not stopped. Patterson recommends the following procedure for stopping this behavior (Patterson, 1975, pp. 118–122).

- *"Re-define what is meant by stealing"* (p. 118). When your child demonstrates a problem with stealing, redefine it as "finding something" and bringing it home, getting into the cookie jar and taking a cookie when told not to do so, or when something looks suspicious and the child could have likely taken it. Explain this new definition to your child. There may be times when your child may be punished for something that she or he did not do, but this is necessary for a few weeks to train the child to stop.

- *Explain the behavior change program to your child.* You might say the following:

  Brian, your mother and I have been concerned for a long time about the amount of stealing you do. From now on, every time you steal, you will be punished. If someone calls our home and even thinks you stole something, we will call it "stealing." If you "find" something, don't bring it home because we will call it "stealing." If we have items missing around the house, and it even looks like you might have stolen it, we will call it "stealing." To avoid being punished for something you didn't do, you need to stay away from things that will look like stealing. (p.120)

- *Make a home contract/point chart with consequences listed.* An example of a point contract (sheet) can be seen in Figure 9.1. If your child has a problem only with lying, you may want to add this to your present point chart or make a point chart/contract for lying only.

After a few weeks, you are likely to find that stealing and/or lying are occurring less frequently. When this happens, *gradually* decrease the number of points that can be earned for "no stealing" and "no lying," and add other behaviors, such as "completing chores," "doing homework." After a few months, you may find that you no longer need the point chart; however, continue with the consequences for stealing or lying if they occur again. It is likely that your child may test you sometime in the future to see if you will still follow through with the consequences.

Point Contract

Behavior (points possible)	M	T	W	Th	F	S	S
No Stealing (4)	4	0	0				
No Lying (2)	2	0	2				
Total	6	0	2				

Consequences: 6 points: 9:00 bedtime, plus a game of Sorry before bed

4 points: 8:30 bedtime

2 points: 8:00 bedtime, plus wash dishes

0 points: 7:30 bedtime, plus wash dishes for two days

Time-out for lying; 1 hour of housework for stealing, plus child returns the item or buys the person a replacement with allowance money

_____   _____   _____   _____
Child's Signature   Date   Parent's Signature   Date

Note. Adapted from *Families: Applications of Social Learning to Family Life* (p. 121), by G. R. Patterson, 1975, Champaign, IL: Research Press. Copyright 1975 by Research Press.

FIGURE 9.1. Sample Point Contract.

If you have followed these approaches to addressing problems with lying and stealing, and they continue to occur at a high rate, it is recommended that you work with a mental health professional to extinguish these behaviors.

? My child will be in a school next year that changes classes. How can I help my child to be more successful in this setting? I worry that she will do poorly.

The transition from a self-contained classroom in an elementary school to one in which the school is departmentalized (e.g., one teacher for math, one for the language arts, one for science, etc.) can be very difficult for some children. Possible areas of concern may result because (1) each teacher has her or his own way of communicating with the students, and the child with ADHD often experiences greater difficulty adjusting to different communication styles; (2) the amount of homework is not easily monitored because the teachers may not communicate daily (for example, one evening your child may have no homework and then the next evening, your child has homework in all subjects); or (3) the child with ADHD is often deficient in organizational and study skills and is not an independent learner, so she or he may experience greater difficulty prioritizing the subjects and completing long-range projects in a timely manner.

During this time, it may be helpful to identify someone to help your child (at least initially) with this transition. It is usually best that this person be someone within the school (see the previous chapter for additional school intervention suggestions). A "coach" can meet daily with your child to make sure that all assignments are listed in the assignment book and that books are gathered that need to be taken home. This person can also serve as a liaison among each of your child's teachers, as well as with your child and you. The use of a coach should be gradually reduced during the school year rather than stopped abruptly. Also, do not hesitate to ask for regular meetings with school personnel. *Gradually* encourage your preadolescent or adolescent to participate in these meetings.

Some parents of students with ADHD have found that there are also advantages to departmentalization. First, many children with ADHD do better with variety. Changing classes will provide your child with more novelty in the school environment. Second, some preadolescents and adolescents can maintain attention for 50 minutes when they know that they will be allowed to move around after class. My son said that changing classes was better because he knew he only had to listen to the teacher for 50 minutes, and then he could go to the hall to talk to his friends. Third, you may have three or four very good teachers and only one poor teacher, whereas when your child has only one teacher for the entire day as in elementary school, you could be unlucky in the teacher selection for the entire year.

Remember that the best policy is to be proactive. Help your child by establishing the homework routine by the first week of school; don't wait until he or she fails a class to do this (see Chapter 8 for guidelines for establishing the homework routine). If this is not enough, schedule a meeting with school personnel to discuss a better communication plan between home and school and establish a home–school incentive program as described in Chapter 8.

? What are some techniques I can use to help my child improve her organizational skills?

First, I would encourage you to model good organizational skills. If your home is a mess and you have difficulty locating items in your home, it is likely that your child will model these skills. Second, begin with one behavior or activity, and establish an organizational plan for it. If you decide to work on keeping a clean room, establish an organizational plan for this—books in one place, toys in the toy box, dirty clothes in the hamper, and so on.

Other possible ways include helping your child set a goal you know she can reach and working on one goal at a time. Build in routines for completing homework and chores at home. Build in a reward incentive program for your child when writing her assignments in the assignment book. This will help to build positive habits. Assist your child (or have a tutor assist) in setting short-term goals for long assignments. Many students with ADHD put off completing assignments until the last minute. Initially, your child will need help with this; then *gradually* reduce the amount of help you are giving her.

Sometimes, you must decide which battle you are going to fight. If there are other, more pressing concerns, you may decide to wait on organizing the bedroom. Don't sweat the small stuff, and pick your battles wisely.

❓ *Due to my child's impulsive behavior (mainly talking), Peter loses special privileges that the entire class receives on Friday. He appears to be the only one who loses these privileges. How can I help him to feel better about himself when he is trying his best? The rule: three interruptions per day results in a lost privilege.*

First, ask for a meeting with the teacher. Don't approach this meeting in an adversarial style, but seek the teacher's assistance in helping your child reach this goal. Arrive at the meeting with an open mind. Ask your child's teacher several questions: What is the definition of an interruption? How many times does Peter interrupt per day? Can you give me daily feedback on the number of interruptions he has each day by sending me a note or putting it on his "Home–School Card"? Is there positive feedback when he does not interrupt? Ensure the teacher that you will support her in your son's efforts to meet the goal. Also, ask the teacher if she feels that your son is capable of reaching this goal.

If his teacher says that your son typically interrupts four or five times per day, then the goal of three per day would be obtainable with appropriate and more immediate incentives. If, however, he is interrupting many more than three times, it is unlikely that he will be able to reach the goal of three or fewer per day without a behavior plan in place in the school and/or at home. (If this is the case, you may need to solicit help from an objective observer.) I worked with one teacher who had a child in her classroom who averaged 126 interruptions per day. To expect this child to reduce his interruptions from 126 to 3 per day would have been an unrealistic expectation. Thus, for this child an individualized behavior change program was implemented, and by the end of 2 months, he was averaging less than 10 interruptions per day. While still not what this teacher expected for the remainder of the class, his improvement was noteworthy.

When you arrive home, ask your child if he can tell you what is meant by an interruption. Role-play with him and then immediately reinforce him when he does not interrupt you or another family member. Give Peter many opportunities for positive practice—for example, "Peter, that was an interruption. How could you have asked me to help you without interrupting my conversation with your dad?" If your son is interrupting 10 times each day, set a goal at home of about 20% below this and reward him for his progress (put this on your point system behaviors). For example, for week one, if

Peter interrupts 8 or fewer times per day, he would earn 5 points on the point chart (or another appropriate reward). Also, remember to provide him with positive feedback. If he consistently meets this goal, lower the goal to 6 or 7 the next week. Gradually lower the number until he is able to reach the goal of 3.

It is my impression that we do not help our children if we just say, "My child cannot meet the goal set for the remainder of the class because he has ADHD." If the goal is reasonable and appropriate, it is better to identify a way to help your child reach this goal. Can you imagine how your child might feel when he reaches this goal? The pride that he will feel in accomplishing this goal will do wonders for his self-esteem.

? *After a good day at school (or camp), where my child is given generous amounts of positive feedback for his behavior, John seems to do everything he can to get into trouble at home. He seems to deliberately want to "self-destruct" a very positive situation when he arrives home.*

There could be a number of reasons for this, as well as a number of possible suggestions for improving this behavior. Some children who are taking a short-acting stimulant (Ritalin or Dexedrine) may experience a rebound. During this rebound time, the child may actually be more hyperactive, moody, and impulsive, and even appear to be worse than before he began taking the medication. For the child who experiences a moderate to severe rebound and when it continues for several weeks after the child has been on medication, a third dose in the late afternoon is sometimes recommended by the prescribing physician. This third dose may help the child complete his homework assignments in a more timely manner, have a more positive evening with the family, and sleep better. The timing and dosage of medication is individual to each child; however, this dose is often smaller (sometimes one-half the dose) than the dose he takes while in school. This smaller dose often helps to reduce or eliminate the rebound some children experience.

It is also helpful to carefully observe the environment. Is the afternoon overly scheduled? Does he have time to unwind after school and just be a child (e.g., ride his bike, shoot baskets)? John may need some time alone before too much is expected of him. Is there a set routine for the family, or is it chaotic and unpredictable? Remember that our children do better when they know what is expected of them and they know the routine. Avoid quizzing your child the moment you pick him up from school. Listen carefully to what he is saying, as well as the feelings beneath the words.

? *How can I help my child understand that she has ADHD and how this affects her behavior?*

There are a number of books and videos available for children that are intended to help them understand the disorder. Some of these are listed in Appendix A. Rebecca Kajander (1995, p. 61) suggests that parents discuss the following with their young children and allow older children to read the information themselves (this information can be shared in many different settings rather than all at one time):

- ADHD is not a disease. It is just the way your brain works.

- When the attention control center in your brain is weak, it is said that you have attention-deficit disorder. Some children have a hard time sitting still and need to move around a lot. This is called being hyperactive.

- You were born with ADHD.

- Having ADHD does not mean you are stupid or dumb. It has nothing to do with how smart you are.

- Having ADHD does not mean you are "bad," but sometimes it is hard to stop and think long enough to make good choices, even if you really want to.

- Some children take medicine to help them. (If your child is taking medication, help her understand why she is taking medication.)

- Taking medication is like wearing glasses. It helps focus your brain, like glasses help to focus your eyes.

- Even though you have ADHD, there are still many things you can do well. Some things will be harder for you, like listening and following directions. Enjoy what you do well, and work hard on those things that are difficult. I will help you!

? *Whom do we tell about ADHD and medication? Should we tell my son's grandparents or parents of his friends? What do we tell them?*

It is often important to share with close friends and family the truth about your child. If they are close friends, they already know that your child is overly active if he has the predominately hyperactive/impulsive type or the combined type of ADHD. They may even be blaming you for his difficulty in controlling his impulsivity and activity level. Share with them the same way you might if your child had diabetes or a learning disability. If your child is taking medication, let them know it is similar to wearing glasses; it helps your child focus better and not be so impulsive. Information can be shared casually when the conversation presents itself. Let them know that your child is getting help and that you would appreciate their support. If you know that your friends or family members will be critical of you for your decision to place your child on medication, you may avoid telling them unless your child needs to take medication while in their home. You can tell them in a matter-of-fact manner

▶ He needs this medication in order to be more successful and have improved behavior in group and social activities. He tends to get overly excited and has greater difficulty controlling his impulsivity and activity level when there is a great deal of stimulation or if there are unclear expectations. He wants to do well, but sometimes it is harder when there is not enough structure.

At some point, your son will be his own advocate and may feel comfortable telling his friends. I have often found that parents of children with ADHD actually have better parenting skills than their friends who have children with "easy" temperaments.

Parents of children with ADHD have demonstrated significant efforts to understand their child and learn good parenting techniques. They often become the experts when their friends are having difficulty with their children. As a result, you may be sought out for advice.

? *Obviously, some people have already been "put off" by my daughter's impulsive, hyper behavior. What can we do to ease things for her in her relationships with peers and their families and to avoid or effectively deal with any concerns they may have?*

There are a number of suggestions that might be helpful to you and your child. Consider the following:

- Before your child is to visit in others' homes or to be in a new situation, review with her the rules for behavior and your expectations. Let the parents know which management approaches work best with your child and which situations are difficult for her. Role-play with your child certain situations before placing her in that environment.

- If friends are visiting in your home, review the family rules before a friend arrives. Keep the activities simple, and it is usually best to invite only one friend at a time. Plan activities as much as possible so your child knows what to expect. She is more likely to remain in control if she knows which activities they will do.

- Never criticize your child in front of her friends.

- Remember that it will be more difficult for your child to remain in control of her behavior in a highly stimulating, unstructured environment. If placed in that situation, you may need a time for the two of you to take a self-control break so she can regain control (e.g., take a quiet walk, look for pebbles in the stream, come in the house for a snack).

With the amount of effort you have put into learning effective parenting strategies, it is quite possible that the friends will notice the change, and you will not need to tell them anything. They may ask you, "What have you done? Rebecca is a different child."

? *How can I get cooperation from other family members, instead of opposition, to implement routines?*

If the lack of cooperation is with your spouse, it can be very difficult for the entire family. If both parents cannot agree on how they will parent a child with ADHD, the child is more likely to split the parents, and the child's progress could be limited. It may be that a compromise is needed. If one parent resists routines, begin by setting one routine such as "getting up in the morning" or "going to bed" for your child. Try the procedure suggested in Chapter 4 of this book. By doing so, it is hoped that the other parent will see the progress your child is making and also see the importance of this procedure.

It is best to avoid disagreeing with your spouse in front of the child. This, too, will split you. Don't give up. Continue doing what you know to be good parenting. Your child may resist now, but she or he will learn who can be trusted to follow through on rewards and consequences. It may also help to occasionally insert a pleasant surprise in your normal routine. You and your child may need a break from the routine. Some days you may need a little novelty to avoid feeling stressed by the same routine each day.

? *How do we handle family members (grandparents, aunts) with whom my child with ADHD spends large amounts of time? Do we ask them to award points and follow our house rules? Should they have their own set of house rules that they enforce?*

If you are visiting in their home, your child must follow their rules, and they will likely be different from the ones you have in your home. Ask them to inform you of their rules within their home so that you can prepare your child. Most homes have a few rules they expect to be followed (e.g., sitting at the dinner table while eating, no running in the house). You can also inform them, for example, that you have been working on Johnny's "back talk" or arguing with adults. While he is in their home, it would be helpful if they would let you know how he is doing with this one behavior. You could ask them to rate this behavior from 1 to 5, with 5 being best. Then you could award points for your child's behavior that was exhibited in their home.

If your child is in others' home almost daily, ask that they decide on the rules for behavior while your child is in their home and to decide on consequences for rule violations. Also, model for them the manner in which you give positive feedback to your child. When you return for your child, you can have the family members rate your child's behavior (e.g., rating from 1 to 5 or the number of times he was in time-out) and then award additional bonus points on the point chart for behavior away from home.

Another approach might be to inform your child ahead of time that you will award a certain number of bonus points for each compliment you receive from your relative concerning her or his behavior while in their home. This approach will be relatively easy for all parties involved.

? *What do you recommend if a behavior such as whining recurs after it has been dropped from the point contract?*

It could recur because it was dropped prematurely from your point system behaviors. Remember that eliminating a long-standing problem that has been a habit for many years cannot be accomplished overnight. The best approach to stop whining is to stop reinforcing the whining and teach the child a more appropriate way of speaking. Most children whine because they get the attention of the parent when they whine. If your child is very young and is just beginning to talk, this approach to stopping whining is not recommended. At a young age, children need a great deal of practice in talking. You do not want to cut off this communication and experimentation with words. This approach could work for children already talking and on into the teen years. You might first try the following:

- When your child speaks to you in a normal tone of voice, stop immediately and listen to her or him if at all possible. If you can't listen at that time, at least acknowledge that you have heard her or him, and state something like, "That sounds really interesting, let me get off the phone, and then you can tell me. I want to hear about it."

- Actively ignore your child when she or he whines (turn your back, read the newspaper, go into another room).

If this approach does not work to eliminate the whining, consider the approach outlined by Howard Sloane (1979, pp. 82–96). He suggests an extended five-step approach. His first step includes the following:

If your child asks for something without whining . . .

A. If possible, grant the request.

B. If it is not possible to grant the request, tell your child why not or when you can grant the request.

C. Thank the child for asking nicely.

If your child whines . . .

D. Without being critical, explain in one sentence how whining makes you feel.

E. Demonstrate a better way to say it.

F. Ask the child to perform correctly if this has not already happened.

G. If the child responds properly, go to parts A, B, and C above.

H. If the child does not respond at all or whines again, tell the child once more to say it properly.

I. If the child then responds properly, go to parts A, B, and C.

J. If the child again does not respond or whines, ignore the child.

K. If the child says it properly, go to parts A, B, and C. (p. 94)

Sloan recommends continuing this step for 4 days and then moving to step 2 if it is needed. Additional suggestions are in his book, *The Good Kid Book*.

❓ How should financial matters (allowance) be handled differently with the children with ADHD (if any difference is necessary)?

The way you handle financial matters will depend, in part, on the age of your child. It is usually a worthwhile experience for children to receive an allowance. It helps them learn to manage their money and to set priorities. Below is an approach used with my children at 10, 14, and 16 years of age. The 14-year-old was the son with ADHD.

▶ Being a single parent, it was frustrating being asked for money each day. I never seemed to have enough to meet all their needs, and I felt that they needed to manage their own money and avoid coming to me each time money was needed. The children were first instructed to detail their financial needs for one month (make a budget). They were to list lunch money, spending money, gas money for the 16-year-old, gift money, and so on. After a careful review, the amount was determined that each child would receive at the beginning of the month. The amount was different for each child. The kids' job was to manage their own money for the month. If Emily wanted to make her lunch for school and save her money, she could do this. If one child had a special event that was not anticipated, she or he could ask if there were additional chores around the house that could be completed to earn money. The girls managed their money well, and Thomas was out of money in 2 weeks. I had to refrain from bailing Thomas out; he needed to experience the consequences of his behavior. He didn't go hungry at school. He either took his lunch or borrowed from his girlfriends.

This was an important lesson for him and for me. Thomas needed more guidance in helping him to manage his money. I also found that one month was too long for Thomas. The next month, I gave him his money on Sunday to last for the week. When he could consistently handle a week, I moved to 2 weeks. By *gradually* increasing the time period, I helped him to be more successful.

? *How can I help my child feel more comfortable speaking with adults?*

Some children are just naturally shy and need time to "warm up" before they feel comfortable talking to adults. This may be your child's temperament, with which she or he was born. Another reason for being uncomfortable or shy with others could be a possible language disorder. Some researchers believe that as many as 50% of children with ADHD have some type of language disorder (Love & Thompson, 1988). It is also suggested that more children with ADHD, predominantly inattentive type, have language disorders than those who have the hyperactive/impulsive type. Many children with language disorders need more time to process auditory information and more time to organize a response.

There are several ways in which you may be helpful, whether your child is "slow-to-warm-up" or has a language disorder.

- Teach your child certain "scripts" to use when she or he meets new people or is placed in a new situation. For example, "Hi, my name is Sally. What's yours?" By learning "scripts," your child may feel more comfortable when meeting new people.

- Prepare your child for a new situation. Talk about what the situation may be like, who might be there, and possible topics of conversation.

- You may need to cue your child in a conversation, but allow her or him as many opportunities as possible to add to the conversation. The more times your child has to practice, the more confident she or he will become.

Often, we speak for the child in an attempt to help. By doing this, we cause the child to lose many opportunities to enhance the conversational skills and her or his feelings of self-worth. If your child does have a language disorder, one good book is *Childhood Speech, Language, and Listening Problems: What Every Parent Should Know*, by Hamaguchi (1995).

? *How can a man learn how to be a better communicator with his child, his child's teacher, and his family?*

First and foremost, a person (whether male or female) must have the desire to be a better communicator. The foundation for good communication skills is to be a good listener. Forgatch and Patterson in their book *Parents and Adolescents Living Together* (1989) suggest eight guidelines for improving listening. These are listed in Chapter 4 of this book. Bruce Baldwin, in *Behind the Cornucopia Kids* (1988, p. 99), lists three actions that shut down parental communication:

- The parent tries to control the conversation.
- The parent focuses on getting information quickly.
- The parent quickly imposes her or his values or judges prematurely.

If each of us could follow the eight guidelines suggested by Forgatch and Patterson for improving listening and communicating with our children or with anyone else (e.g., bosses, other family members, teachers), communication could be greatly improved.

? *How can I move my child to more maturity for his age?*

First, obtain a good book that will provide you with information relative to what is developmentally appropriate for each age. One good book is *You and Your Adolescent: A Parent's Guide for Ages 10–20,* by Steinberg and Levine (1990). In addition, Louise Ames, Frances Ilg, and Sidney Baker have written a series of books on the developmental levels of children. Research has shown that children with ADHD tend to be behind their peers in social maturity, sometimes as much as 2 to 4 years. Because of this, it is critical that your expectations be realistic and that you do not place your child in situations that guarantee failure. As with any other behavior, *gradually* increase your expectations to avoid frustration and loss of self-esteem. A number of suggestions are made in Chapter 7 of this book that may enable your child to grow in his maturity. The suggestions made in regard to locating and cultivating competencies in your child and learning to accept responsibility for behaviors may be particularly helpful.

If your child has social skills deficits, provide him with encouragement and assistance in techniques to build these skills. Talk about ways a situation could have been handled, what the child could have said, and how he can be a good friend. Stage situations at home that will help the child to improve these skills. For example, invite one peer at a time to the home. It would be helpful if this peer would demonstrate positive social behaviors for your child.

? *How do you get after-school care personnel to cooperate when you request assistance with intervention for your child?*

When you turn your child over to others to be her or his caregivers, you also turn over the role of disciplining your child. The after-school setting is different than that found in most schools. You cannot force the after-school providers to follow the suggestions made by other professionals who are working with your child. If the director is unwilling to take the suggestions of your child's therapist or other professionals working with him, you may need to find another option for after-school care. Ask for a meeting with the director and use your good listening techniques. Set up the plan as you would with the school as described in Chapter 8. You can also place some of the after-school care behaviors on your point chart used at home.

❓ *What should I do when an older sibling who has ADHD constantly pushes, hits, or slaps the face of a younger sibling and causes injuries? To make it worse, he then lies about it even when the action was witnessed.*

First, review the lying section presented in this chapter. If you saw the child hit the younger sibling, immediately punish the older child for the aggression. *Do not* ask the child if he did it or why he did it. That places the child in a situation to lie. Also, make sure you are providing the child with ADHD-adequate attention when he appropriately plays or interacts with his sibling. If the only time he gets your attention is after hitting his brother, he will continue to do this. Control any urge you may have to hit the aggressor. Place the child in time-out for the aggression, and do this in as calm a manner as possible. Ask the older sibling to tell you when he is angry with his little brother, rather than hitting him. When he does tell you, respond to his comments. Do not scold him for having these feelings. Accept these feelings as real, even though they may not be accurate. Praise him for verbalizing these feelings rather than hitting his brother.

Structure positive sibling relationships. Help your children find appropriate ways to relate to each other. Also, give the older sibling roles to play with the younger sibling. For example, the older sibling may be placed in the teacher role: "You have been playing ball so well at camp, please take your brother outside and play catch with him." You might also place him in the role of comforter. When the younger sibling is hurt, let the older sibling help take care of him.

In addition, don't always assume that the younger sibling is innocent of everything. There may be times when the younger sibling initiated the fight. You should still punish the aggressive act the same way; just be observant of the younger siblings' actions.

It may also be helpful to have a "cooling off" area for the children. For example, when they appear to be approaching aggression, inform them that one child must go to one side of the yard and the other to the opposite side. They must remain in their own area until they have "cooled off." You do not need to require that they apologize when they have calmed down.

❓ *Is it important for the child with ADHD to keep her environment orderly, bedroom picked up, and so forth?*

Decide what is reasonable for your family. If a messy room is interfering with the child's or your family's daily functioning, the room may need to be kept more orderly. For example, if a messy room results in things being lost or broken, if a sibling shares the room and is annoyed by the mess, or if someone could get hurt, then the room may need to be kept more orderly. Determine what is appropriate based on the child's age. Another important rule is to *never clean the room for your child.* If you clean it, your child will never do it. Follow the guidelines in Chapter 6 for setting up a point chart or a contract.

Some parents find that the best way to resolve the problem of a messy room is to close the child's door (as long as the room does not interfere with the family's functioning as described above). However, it is important that the family area remain uncluttered. Children, as well as their parents, should be responsible for keeping the family area free of their belongings. To assist with this problem, you may provide the family with a large box in which all articles are placed when they are left in the family area at bedtime. For example, if mom leaves her keys on the dining room table, they are thrown in the box. It will take some effort to retrieve these.

? How do I help my child's older siblings get on the bandwagon of positive reinforcement rather than arguing or putting their brother with ADHD down?

You may want to have a family meeting with the older siblings. Discuss with them what you have learned about parenting and the role you would like for them to play in your son's life. If they are angry with him for something he has said or done, encourage them to come to you and share these feelings rather than taking it out on their brother. Teach them appropriate ways to share their concerns or feelings with their brother that do not label him or "put him down."

You may want them to read books such as *My Brother's a World Class Pain: A Sibling's Guide to ADHD/Hyperactivity,* by Michael Gordon; and *Living with ADHD: A Practical Guide to Coping with Attention Deficit Hyperactivity Disorder,* by Rebecca Kajander. Books like these can help siblings to have a better understanding of the disorder and the reasons for their brother's behavior and actions. You will not be making excuses for his behavior, but you will be soliciting their help in helping your son improve.

Also, encourage the family to identify strengths in your son with ADHD and provide him with many opportunities to share and use these strengths. This will get the siblings into the habit of looking for positive qualities in him. Give his siblings positive feedback when they share a positive comment with him.

What Happens When Children Approach the Adolescent Years?

The future belongs to those who believe in the beauty of their dreams.

—Eleanor Roosevelt

Children, whether they have ADHD or not, will likely have a difficult time during the adolescent years. Even the best parents will have some difficulty with their child during the adolescent years just because of the changes that are occurring when a child makes the transition from childhood to adolescence. If you have practiced the principles presented in this book, however, you may find that the adolescent years are not as difficult as you had anticipated. Parents of children with ADHD who have used a balanced parenting plan are better prepared for the adolescent years. While the problems during adolescence will not be eliminated, the foundation will be stronger, and the problems are often managed with greater confidence and less anxiety. This balanced plan of parenting should include the following:

- using proactive strategies in your parenting by establishing routines, structure, and guidelines for your child

- attending to and spending time with your child

- delivering generous amounts of positive reinforcement when you have observed positive behaviors

- consistently using mild forms of punishment for inappropriate behavior

- using powerful motivators when the regular positive feedback and punishment do not work to change inappropriate behavior

- avoiding the tendency to use the ADHD label to excuse inappropriate behavior

- maintaining a sense of humor that allows you and your child to learn from mistakes and to forgive yourself and your child when mistakes are made

What are the normal changes in a child who is approaching adolescence?

Robin and Foster (1989) note that adolescents face a number of tasks, while at the same time they are adjusting to changes in the way they think, in their biological makeup, and in their emotional functioning. In order for adolescents to move forward to become healthy and competent adults, the following, from Robin and Foster (1989) and Conger (1977), must occur:

NOTES

- The adolescent must begin to separate from her or his parents and become independent. This is the adolescent's major job. (Robin & Foster, 1989, pp. 8–9)

- The adolescent must adjust to physical changes in her or his body and to psychological changes involved in sexual maturity.

- The adolescent must develop a system of values and determine her or his own identity.

- She or he must establish an effective social and working relationship with same- and opposite-sex peers.

- The adolescent must begin preparations for a vocation. (Conger, 1977, p. 220)

Many of the problems you may experience with your child are inherent in the typical adolescence. At times, however, the problems during the adolescent years can be exacerbated because of the symptoms of ADHD. Thus, it is critical that you have a good understanding of what to expect during the adolescent years. This will help you to address specific concerns you might encounter with your adolescent who has ADHD. An excellent resource for all parents whose child is approaching or in the adolescent years is a book written by Laurence Steinberg and Ann Levine, *You and Your Adolescent: A Parent's Guide for Ages 10–20.* Steinberg and Levine suggest that parents can expect some or all of the following to occur during the adolescent years (pp. 151–153):

- "Adolescents will see being close to, or reliant on, their parents as 'babyish'" (p. 151). This may be demonstrated in the way in which they want you to show them affection to a rejection of your offer to help them complete a task.

- "Teenagers don't want to be seen with their parents" (p. 151). Most of the time this occurs because they want to be seen as more independent.

- They have a need for emotional and physical privacy. This too is a way of demonstrating emotional independence. It doesn't always mean they have something to hide.

- Adolescents may try to identify your personal weaknesses and use them against you.

- Friends are often chosen over family. This does not mean that she or he is rejecting the family, but that you are not her or his total world anymore.

- Teens can turn ordinary events or decisions into tests of their competence and your trust. For example, John may have always done his homework before dinner, but now he no longer wants to do it at this time. This may be his way of letting you know that he thinks he is mature enough to make some of his own decisions.

❓ Will the adolescent who has ADHD encounter greater difficulty than other teens?

Since the adolescent's primary job is to gain independence from the family, the adolescent with ADHD may encounter additional obstacles. For example, it has been noted that children with ADHD are not as mature as others who do not have the diagnosis of ADHD. Thus, they often experience greater difficulty making good decisions and weighing the consequences before acting. It should be noted that there is data to suggest that there is a small percentage of adolescents who received a diagnosis of ADHD in childhood who will not manifest the symptoms that would continue to warrant a diagnosis in adolescence (Goldstein, 1993). There are, however, a high percentage who will continue to demonstrate sufficient symptoms into the adolescent years. The symptoms may change somewhat, but nevertheless, they continue to affect the adjustment of the adolescent. For example, Weiss and Hechtman (1986) found that teens with ADHD may not be as overactive as they were as children, but that impulsivity and inattention continue to be problematic. For example, my son as a high school student was not as fidgety, but he received several speeding tickets because of his impatience and impulsivity.

The adolescent years are not hopeless just because your teen has ADHD. If you go into the adolescent years with as much information as possible, you can survive these years, and you might even enjoy them. Arthur Robin suggests that parents of teens with ADHD consider the following in their parenting (Barkley, 1995, p. 189):

- First, understand adolescent development and the impact of ADHD on it.

- Develop strategies for coping with your adolescent.

- Determine reasonable expectations. For example, it may be unrealistic for you to expect your teen to make all A's in school; however, it might be realistic for your child to make A's and B's. For some teens C's are reasonable because of other conditions the teen might have. It may also be unrealistic for your teen to keep her or his room clean; however, a realistic expectation might be that the room be cleaned at least one time per week. If you have some unrealistic expectations, discuss these with your spouse or a neutral party to assist in setting more realistic goals.

- Establish, monitor, and enforce appropriate house and street rules. Develop these with your teen's input.

- Continue to communicate positively and use good communication strategies (e.g., "I messages" rather than "you messages"; use good listening techniques as discussed in Chapter 4).

- Use effective problem-solving strategies with your teen (review Chapter 7 for the STPDE plan).

- If professional help is needed, carefully seek it from someone who understands adolescent development as well as ADHD.

- Maintain a sense of humor with your teen and spouse.

- Take regular vacations from your teen.

There are many joys in parenting a teen with ADHD, and you will have many funny stories to tell your friends and families (in later years). Of course, it is much easier for one to identify these as "funny" when the teen has left the house than when you are in the midst of these years. Despite the joys, there are areas to carefully consider before your teen reaches these events. These are discussed below.

Driving

Many teens with ADHD are not ready to drive the day they turn 16 years of age. In addition, it is not advisable to buy your teen the fastest and most powerful sports car on the day she or he turns 16. The teen with ADHD is not ready for this responsibility. If your state does not have a "graduated" license, develop a plan with your teen to prepare him or her for this responsibility. Consider developing this contract one year prior to her or his sixteenth birthday. The contract could cover several of the following issues:

- A great deal of supervised practice time with adults is important. This could include 350 hours of practice time with her or his parents before obtaining a driver's license. *Make* your teen drive you to the store, to church, and to work in order that she or he can acquire as much practice as possible. Some of this time should be at night.

- After these hours have been logged and driver's education classes have been taken, your teen may be ready for a probationary license. As a condition of the probationary license, your teen must drive for 3 months with no accidents (that were her or his fault) or tickets before she or he is ready for the next level of license. During those first 3 months, consider including a statement that only one other teen is allowed in the car with her or him, and she or he must be home before dark.

- If your teen has successfully met the criteria for the first 3 months of probation, then you can gradually extend the privileges (e.g., driving at night, no more than two people in the car). The key is to gradually extend the freedom as your teen assumes greater responsibility and has more practice time.

- After 6 months of accident-free (not her or his fault) and ticket-free driving, your teen has earned the right to have additional responsibilities with the car.

Unsupervised Times

Police records indicate that most teen crimes occur immediately after school and before dark. This occurs because this time is usually unsupervised and unstructured. Thus, your teen will continue to need monitoring during these unstructured times of day. If your teen is involved in after-school sports or another activity, fewer incidents involving crime are likely to occur. If your teen is not involved in after-school sports, you may require that your teen be involved in other activities outside of school (e.g., job for two hours after school, Tae Kwon Do lessons, working with younger children at a boys' or girls' club). If you work outside the home, you may consider including the following in your house rules: "Call Mother or Father at work when you arrive home from school," and "Before any guests can be invited into the home when parents are not home, permission must be obtained."

Dating and Sexual Activities

Educate your teen. Don't expect that she or he knows all the answers. Talk about the risks of getting pregnant and how the teen's impulsivity may result in an unwanted pregnancy. Talk about AIDS and sexually transmitted diseases. You may also include several rules related to dating in your house rules (e.g., "Inform the family of where you are and who you are with"—this is for both parents and teens).

School Performance

There are a number of reasons for problems in school. These may include the following:

- It becomes more difficult to communicate with teachers when your child is in high school. This may be due to the increase in the number of teachers your teen has, but part of it is due to your teen's reluctance to have you communicate with the teachers. Remember that the adolescent's primary job is to individuate from her or his parents. Your adolescent thinks she or he can handle everything alone.

- Another reason school problems may surface is that many teens with ADHD adopt a passive approach to learning. They tend to do only what they think is required but spend very little time actively thinking about what they are doing. They view other things, such as dating, peers, and cars, as more important.

- Many teens with ADHD experience difficulty with organization, time management, note taking, and completing lengthy written assignments. Some of the strategies suggested in Chapter 8 would be appropriate for the teen (e.g., Weekly Goal Contracts, homework routine, note-taking instruction and strategies, assignment book, medication, and the use of coaches or case managers). If your teen is receiving special education services under IDEA, a transition plan should also be developed (see Chapter 8).

Career Planning

Although this is a part of the Transition Plan for teens who have an IEP, most of the teens who have ADHD do not receive special education services. Thus, most of this responsibility is left to you. Talk to your teen about what she or he likes to do and discuss careers that may use her or his special talents. If your teen did well in school, it is certainly realistic for her or him to go to college. Other teens need more time to mature before going to college. If your teen wants to attend college, work with a college placement counselor in order that an appropriate school can be selected based on your teen's needs, talents, and desires. It is likely that your adolescent will need a coach to work with her or him initially while adjusting from the structure of the home to the less structured college life. Hopefully, your teen will be ready to be her or his own advocate in the postsecondary setting. Some students do better initially in a community college for the first 2 years and then transfer into a 4-year university after making the initial adjustment to college life. Some individuals are not ready for college and do not want to take this route. They may decide later to go to college, but school has been so negative that they need to experience something else. Some teens have elected to join military service and have done extremely well in this setting. Others have worked for a few years and then made the decision to attend college. Give your teen time; she or he should not be forced to complete college in four years.

Teen Forums

Some teens have become involved in support groups for teens with ADHD. These have been helpful in the acceptance of the disorder and in identifying strategies to aid the teen. Your teen may identify an older buddy in one of these support groups, and this person may have greater influence on your teen than you can.

 ### *What can I do now to help increase the chance that my child will become a well-adjusted adult?*

Some of the factors that indicate a better prognosis cannot be changed. For example, it has been reported that children who have a higher IQ, those who have a parent with a higher socioeconomic status, and those whose parents do not have a serious psychiatric disorder have a better prognosis. There are other factors, however, that can contribute to a better adjustment later in life. William Jenson (1995) reports on the research from Robin, Walker, and Patterson and Ekman and Weis and suggests that the following factors may help to improve the prognosis of children with ADHD:

- Those who have good basic reading skills have a better prognosis.

- Those who are argumentative, noncompliant, and aggressive will have greater difficulty as adults. This presents the need for good child-management skills to be consistently implemented.

- Children and adolescents with social skill deficits have greater difficulty as adults. This points to the need for treatment of these deficits.

- Children with ADHD require more supervision; thus, a better prognosis occurs with better monitoring (e.g., having the child or teen call when arriving home and knowing where she or he is).

- When school experiences are linked to employment, the prognosis is better.

- A child who is retained in a grade level, even one time, is more likely to drop out of school. "A widely quoted finding from the Youth in Transition Study is that one grade retention increases the risk of dropping out by 40% to 50%, and being two grades behind increases the risk by 90%" (Bachman, Green, & Wirtanen, 1971).

Sam Goldstein (1993, p. 8) wrote that he is convinced

> that the best predictor of outcome of ADHD in adolescence is not medicine, therapy or educational intervention but rather family variables. Parents accepting of their ADHD adolescent, able to develop a close, positive relationship, capable of being proud, patient and persistent when dealing with school and community resources, and are truly accepting of this human being provide critical insulation and greatly increase the potential for successful adulthood.

Although there are some variables in your child that cannot be changed, such as the child's IQ or the fact that your child has ADHD, you are able to change the way in which you interact with your child or adolescent. In other words, don't worry about the things you cannot change, and focus your time and energy on those variables that you can control.

Final Notes

Parenting is the most important occupation you will ever have. It is also often the most difficult and one for which you are given very little training. Until I was a parent, I did not realize the enormous amount of energy and effort it would take. After I had my first child, I thought parenting was a breeze. Julie was a very easy child to parent. She actually raised herself. She was the "easy child" described earlier. Then, when Thomas was born, I quickly realized that parenting was not as easy as it had been with Julie. He was my "difficult child." At this time, I gained great empathy for others who were parents. I gained new insight into Helen Keller's statement: "Character cannot be developed in ease and quiet. Only through experiences of trial and suffering can the soul be strengthened, vision cleared, ambition inspired and success achieved" (Canfield & Hansen, 1995, p. 272). As parents of children with ADHD, we have tremendous opportunities to build character because it is rare that we experience "ease and quiet." Below are some of the survival tips that have helped me to thrive as a parent.

- If you have a spouse, work together with her or him. If you do not have a spouse, identify a friend who can provide you with support. Share your frustrations and successes with this person.

- If you disagree with your spouse, don't air this disagreement in front of your child. Wait to discuss it in private.

- Plan time to be with your spouse alone. The divorce and separation rate among spouses is higher in families in which children require significant effort to parent.

- Maintain a balance in your life. If your life is stressed because all your time is spent at work or at home parenting the children, you need a better balance in your activities. To maintain a proper balance, you will need time to improve your physical well-being (exercise, enough sleep, eating well-balanced meals), the social–emotional aspects of your life (time with your spouse, friends, etc.), your *spiritual* growth, and your mental development (taking a class, developing a new hobby, reading). Parents, particularly mothers, who assume responsibility for their family's happiness tend to experience greater stress. They may feel drained because they are giving and not receiving anything in return.

- Remember that you deny your children a sense of self-respect when you do everything for them. Children also need to assume some of the responsibility in the home, not only with chores but also with their own happiness.

- Spend time with people who have a positive outlook on life, and maintain your sense of humor. Avoid being around people who are overly negative or critical.

- Look at all the gains your child has made in the last year. The steps may be small, but your child undoubtedly is making progress. Abraham Lincoln is quoted as saying, "We can complain because rose bushes have thorns, or rejoice because thorn bushes have roses." Stop for a few minutes and rejoice in all the gains your child has made over the last year.

My mother taught me very early to believe I could achieve any accomplishment
I wanted to. The first was to walk without braces.

—Wilma Rudolph

Resources

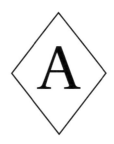

Organizations

ADDA
(National Attention Deficit
Disorder Association)
800-487-2282

ADDult Support Network
c/o Mary Jane Johnson
2620 Ivy Place
Toledo, OH 43613

*American Speech-Language-Hearing
Association* (ASHA)
10801 Rockville Rd.
Rockville, MD 20852
Consumer Helpline: 800-638-8255
http://www.asha.org

Autism Research Institute
4182 Adams Ave.
San Diego, CA 92116
619-281-7165
(primarily devoted to conducting research
on methods of preventing, diagnosing, and
treating autism and other severe behavioral disorders of childhood)

CHADD
(Children & Adults with
Attention Deficit Disorder)
499 NW 70th Ave.
Plantation, FL 33317
305-587-3700.

*Coordinating Council for
Handicapped Children*
220 S. State Street, Room 412
Chicago, IL 60604
(publishes information on advocacy
for parents of children with
developmental disabilities)

Council for Exceptional Children (CEC)
1920 Association Drive
Reston, VA 22091-1589
703-620-3660

Council for Learning Disabilities (CLD)
P.O. Box 40303
Overland Park, KS 66204
913-492-8755

*Learning Disabilities Association of
America* (LDA)
4156 Library Road
Pittsburgh, PA 15234
412-341-1515

*National Adult Literacy and Learning Disabili-
ties Center* (National ALLD Center)
c/o Academy for Educational Development
1875 Connecticut Ave. NW, Suite 800
Washington, DC 20009-1202
202-884-8185

*National Association for Gifted
Children* (NAGC)
115 15th Street NW, Suite 1002
Washington, DC 20005
202-785-4268

*National Center for Youth
with Disabilities*
University of Minnesota
Box 721, 420 Delaware Street SE
Minneapolis, MN 55455
612-626-2825

National Easter Seal Society
230 West Monroe Street, Suite 1800
Chicago, IL 60606
312-726-6200 or 800-221-6827
(runs an information clearinghouse on a
variety of developmental disabilities; also has
a directory of summer programs and short-
term camps for children with special needs)

*National Information Center for Children and
Youth with Disabilities* (NICHCY)
P.O. Box 1492
Washington, DC 20013-1492
800-695-0285
(provides free information to assist parents, educators, caregivers, advocates, and
others in helping children and youth with

disabilities become participating members of the school and community)

National Homeschool Association (NHA)
P.O. Box 157290
Cincinnati, OH 45215-7290
513-772-9580
(a nonprofit membership organization that provides a $3.00 information packet with state support groups and names of relevant magazines, books, and organizations for homeschooling)

PADDA, Peninsula Attention Deficit Disorder Association
12388 Warwick Blvd., Suite 304
Newport News, VA 23606
804-591-9119

The Rebus Institute
1499 Bayshore Blvd., Suite 146
Burlingame, CA 94010
415-697-7424
(a national nonprofit research institute devoted to the study and dissemination of information on adult issues related to ADD and LD through conferences and newsletters)

Federal Laws Affecting Those with Disabilities

P.L. 101-476, Individuals with Disabilities Education Act of 1990 (IDEA). This law replaced the landmark disabilities law PL 94-142, the Education for All Handicapped Children Act of 1975 (EHA). IDEA mandates a free and appropriate public education for all children with disabilities, in the least restrictive environment.

P.L. 102-119, Individuals with Disabilities Education Act of 1991. This law addresses the preschool child with disabilities and amends Part H of the EHA Amendments of 1986. It establishes early intervention programs for children with developmental delays, age birth to 5 years

P.L. 93-112, Rehabilitation Act of 1973 (amended by four other public laws). This law primarily serves adults and youth transitioning into employment settings. Its goal is to develop and implement a comprehensive and coordinated program of vocational assistance and independent living for individuals with disabilities to max-imize their employability and integration into the community.

Section 504 of the Rehabilitation Act, is a civil rights law especially for parents seeking services and school accommodations for their children with disabilities.

P.L. 101-336, Americans with Disabilities Act of 1990 (ADA). This law guarantees equal opportunity for individuals with disabilities in employment, public accommodations, transportation, telecommunication, and state and local government services. It mandates "reasonable accommodations" for all individuals with disabilities.

P.L. 103-227, Goals 2000: Educate America Act (1994). This law establishes a new framework for the federal government to provide assistance to states to reform educational programs to meet today's higher demands. It establishes eight National Education Goals for all children.

P.L. 89-10, Elementary and Secondary Education Act of 1965 (amended by seven other public laws). This law represents the first federal commitment to the improvement of education. It authorized a multibillion-dollar aid program to assist states in educating children from low-income families who were considered educationally disadvantaged (see, Chapter 1).

Newsletters and Handouts

ADDendum (for adults with ADD)
c/o CPS, 5041 Back Lick Road
Annandale, VA 22003
914-278-3022

ADDult News
2620 Ivy Place
Toledo, OH 43613

ADDvisor Attention Deficit Disorder Resource Center
P.O. Box 71223
Marietta, GA 30007-1223

Challenge
P.O. Box 488
West Newbury, MA 01985

MAAP (More Able Austic People)
P.O. Box 524
Crown Point, Indiana 46307
219-662-1311

Journals and Magazines

Adoptive Families
Adoptive Families of America
3333 Highway 100 North
Minneapolis, MN 55422
800-372-3300

Attention!, Published by Ch.A.D.D.
499 NW 70th Ave., Suite 109
Plantation, Florida 33317
305-587-3700
(a magazine for children and adults with attention-deficit disorder)

Journal of Learning Disabilities, Journal of Emotional and Behavioral Disorders, Intervention in School and Clinic, The Journal of Special Education, Topics in Early Childhood Special Education, and *Remedial and Special Education*
published by
PRO-ED
8700 Shoal Creek Boulevard
Austin, TX 78757
512-451-3246

LD Forum and *Learning Disabilities Quarterly*
Publications of the Council for Learning Disabilities, Council for Learning Disabilities
P.O. Box 40303
Overland Park, KS 66204
913-492-8755

Phi Delta KAPPAN
published by Phi Delta Kappa, Inc.
408 N. Union
P.O. Box 789
Bloomington, IN 47402
(an educational journal on a variety of concerns related to public education)

TheirWorld
381 Park Avenue South, Suite 1420
New York, NY 10016
212-545-7510
(a publication of the National Center for Learning Disabilities)

Books for Parents

Barkley, R. A. (1995). *Taking charge of ADHD: The complete authoritative guide for parents.* New York: Guilford Press.

Clark, L. (1989). *The time-out solution: A parent's guide for handling everyday behavior problems.* Chicago–New York: Contemporary Books.

Forgatch, M., & Patterson, G. (1987). *Parents and adolescents living together,* Part 1: *The basics;* Part 2: *Family problem solving.* Eugene, OR: Castalia.

Hamaguchi, P. (1995). *Childhood speech, language, and listening problems: What every parent should know.* New York: John Wiley and Sons.

Kajander, R. (1995). *Living with ADHD: A practical guide to coping with attention deficit hyperactivity disorder.* Minneapolis, MN: Park Nicollet Medical Foundation.

Lelewer, N. (1994). *Something's not right: One family's struggle with learning disabilities.* Acton, MA: VanderWyk & Barnham, a Division of Publicom, Inc.

Steinberg, L., & Levine, A. (1990). *You and your adolescent: A parent's guide for ages 10–20.* New York: Harper Perennial.

Books for Children

Fisher, G., & Commings, R. (1991). *The survival guide for kids with LD.* Minneapolis, MN: Free Spirit Publishing (for children in Grades 2–12).

Galvin, M. (1988). *Otto learns about his medicine: A story about medication for hyperactive children.* New York: Magination Press (for children between the ages of 5 and 10).

Gehret, J. (1990). *Learning disabilities and the don't give up kid.* Fairport, NY: Verbal Images Press (for children in grades 1–3).

Jonover, C. (1988). *Josh, a boy with dyslexia.* Burlington, VT: Waterfront Books (for children in Grades 2–5).

Nadeau, K. G., Dixon, E. B., & Biggs, S. (1993). *School strategies for ADD teens.* Annandale, VA: Chesapeake Psychological Publication.

Videos

Gifts of greatness. Educators Publishing Services, 212-225-5750. An inspiring 1-hour musical drama video highlighting the lives of great people who overcame dyslexia.

Goldstein, S., & Goldstein, M. (1991). *It's just attention disorder. A video for kids.* Neurology, Learning and Behavior Center.

Lavoie, R. (1989). *How difficult can this be?* F.A.T. City, CACLD 203-838-5010 (a video for professionals working with children with a learning disability).

Procedures for Parent Training and Reproducible Sheets

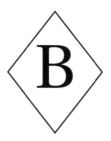

Procedures for Parent Training

Material in this book can be used in an 8- to 10-session parent training course for parents of children between the ages of 5 and 11 years who have ADHD or other disruptive behavior disorders. The information presented in this book is based on the belief that parents can learn to identify their child's strengths and weaknesses and acquire the skills to develop a positive, healthy relationship with their child. Frequently, parents of children with ADHD or other disruptive behaviors may enter the course with inadequate feelings of their own self-worth or of their parenting skills because of their child's disruptive behaviors. Objectives for a parent training course may include the following:

- to equip the parent with skills that will improve his or her confidence level

- to reduce stress within the home

- to improve the child's behavior as well as the parent's response to the child's behavior

- to increase positive habits within the home

- to reduce the rate of inappropriate behaviors exhibited by the child

- to improve the child's compliance rate with authority figures

- to improve the relationship between the child and his or her siblings and between the parent and the child

The course has an educational focus, and it is not meant to be psychotherapy. Most of the parents who attend parent classes and follow the procedures outlined in this book will be able to do what is suggested. There may be a small number, however, who may be unable to make the changes suggested and should be referred to a psychotherapist to provide more intensive intervention.

LEADERS

Leaders for these parent training groups should direct the learning; however, greater learning appears to occur when parents are actively involved and form a supportive network with others in the group. Leaders should have an understanding of ADHD, group dynamics, behavior management, teaching skills, and basic parenting techniques. It may also be beneficial for one leader to be a parent of a child with ADHD. The groups could be led by one or two individuals; however, two leaders are preferred.

FOCUS OF TRAINING

The principles upon which the lessons are based do not represent a cure for ADHD. They are, however, beneficial to the parents in learning to manage the disorder. There is no "magic pill" that will eliminate the problems associated with ADHD. Parents are introduced to strategies that will increase the child's compliance rate, increase the rate of positive behaviors within the home and the school, and improve the relationship between siblings and between parent and child. Because behavior changes slowly, the support and encouragement that occur in this parenting network will help the participants maintain a high level of motivation to continue these strategies even when it appears that little progress is being made. The focus of training is on practical applications, not on theory or a great deal of data collection. Some data collection is suggested at times; however, the parents need to see its practical application.

LOGISTICAL ISSUES

The sessions can be conducted in schools, mental health settings, churches, or community centers. Outcomes of the training are generally more successful in a community-based site, rather than a hospital site or one that is outside the parents' community. Identify a suitable location with facilities that will be conducive to group discussion. Chairs with circular tables that can seat five to eight participants at each table will help to facilitate group exchange. The training can be taught in groups (which is preferred) or individually. It is usually recommended that groups range from 10 to 25 participants. If you offer childcare, arrange for a site that will have a room or gym for appropriate child-centered activities.

TIME GUIDELINES

A 1½- to 2-hour session is usually effective because it allows for a social and networking time prior to the meeting. If you feel this is helpful, plan to have coffee and cookies (or some other snack) prior to each session.

MATERIALS

Flip charts or marking boards are needed for small-group activities (e.g., developing a routine, point system, or contract). In addition, each parent should have a copy of this book. Additional reference books are listed in Appendix A. These materials may be helpful to the leader planning the activities for the week; however, they are not essential. Registration forms are also helpful when enrolling parents in these sessions. Subgroups can be prearranged based on information provided in the registration form (e.g., age of child, primary concerns).

CHILDCARE

Since many parents have difficulty securing childcare, a higher attendance rate is usually maintained when childcare is provided on site. Activities during childcare need to be well organized, with incentives provided to children who follow the rules for appropriate behavior. Rules and consequences need to be clearly specified during the first session. Leaders of the children's groups should practice the principles presented in this book. It has also been helpful for the childcare leader to participate in one of the parent training groups prior to working in the program. One adult should organize the activities and others (e.g., teens, college students wanting experience working with children) assist her or him. It may be possible to obtain volunteers from local colleges and universities. Appropriate activities might include painting, watching a video, playing ball, and reading a book. The last activity of the evening should be a passive, quiet activity, such as listening to a story, in order that the children leave with their parents in a controlled manner.

SOCIAL ACTIVITIES

Organize the parent training sessions to allow for opportunities for positive social interaction with other parents who are experiencing similar problems. Plan a potluck dinner about midway through the training.

FEES

Make the training cost effective. If there are parents who want to attend but who do not have the financial resources, investigate ways to offer scholarships.

ATTENDANCE

Have a method of maintaining attendance records. Stress the importance of both parents attending the training. If parents disagree on the parenting techniques (particularly in front of the child), the child will learn very quickly to manipulate the parents. Because there may be participants who are single parents, provide incentives for single parents to bring a friend or relative to the sessions. It is helpful for each parent to identify another person to support and encourage him or her in using the techniques presented in this book.

INTERACTION TECHNIQUES

Use humor while leading the groups. As a leader, be willing to disclose your failures and successes with your own children. Avoid using technical language, and make your suggestions practical.

HOMEWORK ASSIGNMENTS

Each week, encourage the parents to put into practice the lesson discussed during the session. Occasionally, you may assign parents activities to try at home to address a specific problem they have with their child. This can be an integral part of training because the problems they encounter at home can be discussed during the following meeting.

INFORMATION ON ADHD AND MEDICATION

Because parents will be entering these sessions with different backgrounds and varying levels of understanding of ADHD, the leaders should decide whether a session is needed on the disorder and on medication issues. See Chapter 1 for information on ADHD. A physician or other knowledgeable professional can lead an extra session on the topic of ADHD and medication issues if needed.

EVALUATIONS

Pre- and post-tests are available in this appendix.

Parent Training Registration Form

Participant's Name: _____

Address: _____

Telephone: (W) _____ (H) _____ Training Location: _____

Place of Employment: _____

Name of Child(ren)	Age	Grade	School	List any Diagnoses (ADHD, LD, etc.)

Names of other individual(s) attending course with participant:

Name	Relationship
_____	_____
_____	_____
_____	_____

Parent Training Attendance Sheet

Group Leaders: _____   Dates: _____

Location of Parent Training: _____

Name Relationship	1	2	3	4	5	6	7	8
1.								
2.								
3.								
4.								
5.								
6.								
7.								
8.								
9.								
10.								
11.								
12.								
13.								
14.								
15.								
16.								
17.								
18.								
19.								
20.								
21.								
22.								
23.								
24.								
25.								

Children's Attendance Roll

Session Dates: _____

Group Leader(s): _____

Location: _____

Child's Name	Age/Grade	1	2	3	4	5	6	7	8
1.									
2.									
3.									
4.									
5.									
6.									
7.									
8.									
9.									
10.									
11.									
12.									
13.									
14.									
15.									
16.									
17.									
18.									
19.									
20.									
21.									
22.									
23.									
24.									
25.									

Parent Questionnaire For Parent Training Classes

Pre-Test

Name: _____   Date: _____

Relationship to Child: _____   Child's Grade: _____

Training Location: _____   Child's Age: _____

Please respond to the following areas by circling the number on the scale that corresponds to how you feel about each statement.

0 = None   1 = Rarely or Little   2 = Average or Some   3 = Often or Much   4 = Very Often or Very Much

1. Rate how often you have positive interactions with your child on a daily basis.   0 1 2 3 4

2. Rate how often your child does what you ask the first time you ask him or her.   0 1 2 3 4

3. Rate the amount of individual time you spend each day with your child.   0 1 2 3 4

4. Rate how often your child follows routines each day without reminders (e.g., getting dressed in the morning, going to bed).   0 1 2 3 4

5. Rate how often your child follows your "house rules."   0 1 2 3 4

6. Rate how often your child has positive relations with her or his peers.   0 1 2 3 4

7. Rate how often your child has positive relations with a sister or brother.   0 1 2 3 4

8. Rate how often your child is cooperative at home.   0 1 2 3 4

9. Rate how confident you are in your parenting.   0 1 2 3 4

10. Rate how effective you think your discipline is with your child.   0 1 2 3 4

11. Rate how often your child behaves appropriately when in public places.   0 1 2 3 4

12. Rate how often your child behaves appropriately with the babysitter.   0 1 2 3 4

13. Rate how often you and your spouse agree on the way you should parent your child.   0 1 2 3 4

14. Rate how consistent you are in disciplining your child.   0 1 2 3 4

15. Rate how often your child argues or "talks back" to you.   0 1 2 3 4

16. Rate your level of personal stress.   0 1 2 3 4

17. Rate the level of stress for the entire family.   0 1 2 3 4

18. Rate how often your child is aggressive to others.   0 1 2 3 4

19. Rate how often you spank your child.   0 1 2 3 4

20. Rate how often you yell or shout at your child.   0 1 2 3 4

21. Medication History:

- Is your child currently taking medication for symptoms associated with ADHD or other behavioral or emotional concerns?   ☐ yes   ☐ no

- If yes, why is she or he taking the medication? _____

_____

- Check below the person who is managing or monitoring your child's medication.

    ☐ Pediatrician   ☐ Family Practice Physician

    ☐ Psychiatrist   ☐ Pediatric Neurologist

    ☐ Other _____

- If your child is taking medication, please complete the following:

Name of Medication _____ Dose _____

How many times each day does she or he take this medication? _____

How many years (months) has he or she taken this medication? _____

Has he or she ever taken other medications for this condition?   ☐ yes   ☐ no

What were the names of the other medications? _____

_____

How many years (months) has he or she taken these medications? _____

22. Check other forms of treatment (intervention) you and/or your child have undergone to address his or her problem behaviors and/or emotional concerns.

    ☐ Individual counseling for child   ☐ Family counseling

    ☐ Behavioral management classes   ☐ Individual tutoring

    ☐ Parenting classes   ☐ Social skills group for child

    ☐ Extra help at school   ☐ Other _____

23. Indicate below if your child has been diagnosed with any of the following:

    ☐ Learning disability   ☐ Language disorder   ☐ Oppositional defiant disorder

    ☐ Conduct disorder   ☐ Anxiety disorder   ☐ Attention-deficit disorder

    ☐ Seizures   ☐ Tic disorder   ☐ Health problem _____

Parent Questionnaire For Parent Training Classes

Post-Test

Name: _____ Date: _____

Relationship to Child: _____ Child's Grade: _____

Training Location: _____ Child's Age: _____

Please respond to the following areas by circling the number on the scale that corresponds to how you feel about each statement.

0 = None   1 = Rarely or Little   2 = Average or Some   3 = Often or Much   4 = Very Often or Very Much

1. Rate how often you have positive interactions with your child on a daily basis.   0 1 2 3 4

2. Rate how often your child does what you ask the first time you ask him or her.   0 1 2 3 4

3. Rate the amount of individual time you spend each day with your child.   0 1 2 3 4

4. Rate how often your child follows routines each day without reminders
    (e.g., getting dressed in the morning, going to bed).   0 1 2 3 4

5. Rate how often your child follows your "house rules."   0 1 2 3 4

6. Rate how often your child has positive relations with his or her peers.   0 1 2 3 4

7. Rate how often your child has positive relations with a sister or brother.   0 1 2 3 4

8. Rate how often your child is cooperative at home.   0 1 2 3 4

9. Rate how confident you are in your parenting.   0 1 2 3 4

10. Rate how effective you think your discipline is with your child.   0 1 2 3 4

11. Rate how often your child behaves appropriately when in public places.   0 1 2 3 4

12. Rate how often your child behaves appropriately with the babysitter.   0 1 2 3 4

13. Rate how often you and your spouse agree on the way you should parent your child.   0 1 2 3 4

14. Rate how consistent you are in disciplining your child.   0 1 2 3 4

15. Rate how often your child argues or "talks back" to you.   0 1 2 3 4

16. Rate your level of personal stress.   0 1 2 3 4

17. Rate the level of stress for the entire family.   0 1 2 3 4

18. Rate how often your child is aggressive to others.   0 1 2 3 4

19. Rate how often you spank your child.   0 1 2 3 4

20. Rate how often you yell or shout at your child.   0 1 2 3 4

21. What did you find the most helpful in the parenting classes? _____

_____

_____

_____

22. What did you find the least helpful? _____

_____

_____

_____

23. What suggestions would you make to improve the training? _____

_____

_____

_____

24. Was the length of the sessions adequate to meet your needs?

    Number of weeks? ☐ yes   ☐ no

    Number of hours each week? ☐ yes   ☐ no

25. Did both parents attend? ☐ yes   ☐ no

26. What portion of your homework assignments did you complete?

    ☐ all   ☐ some   ☐ none

27. What portion of the parenting book have you read?

    ☐ all   ☐ some   ☐ none

28. Would you recommend this class to other parents? ☐ yes   ☐ no

Reproducible Charts

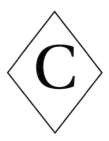

Monitoring Compliance

Date: _____ Beginning Time: _____ Ending Time: _____

Person giving commands: _____

Circle "yes" if your child complied with your command within 5 seconds of your giving it. Circle "no" if your child did not comply within the first 5 seconds of your giving the command.

1. yes	no	11. yes	no
2. yes	no	12. yes	no
3. yes	no	13. yes	no
4. yes	no	14. yes	no
5. yes	no	15. yes	no
6. yes	no	16. yes	no
7. yes	no	17. yes	no
8. yes	no	18. yes	no
9. yes	no	19. yes	no
10. yes	no	20. yes	no

Number of commands given: _____

Number of minutes monitored: _____

Average number of commands given in 1 hour: _____

Compliance rate (divide the number of times your child complied within 5 seconds by the number of commands given):

_____

House Rules

1.

2.

3.

4.

5.

6.

7.

8.

9.

10.

We agree to abide by the rules established in our family meeting on _____.

Date

_____   _____
Parent's Signature   Parent's Signature

_____   _____
Child's Signature   Child's Signature

_____   _____
Other Signature   Other Signature

Behavior Tracking Card

Behavior to increase: _____

_____

Behavior to decrease: _____

_____

Behaviors	Day _____ Time _____	Day _____ Time _____	Day _____ Time _____	Day _____ Time _____
Behavior to Increase _____ _____	Rate: _____	Rate: _____	Rate: _____	Rate: _____
Behavior to Decrease _____ _____	Rate: _____	Rate: _____	Rate: _____	Rate: _____

Rate for positive behavior: _____

Rate for inappropriate behavior: _____

Contract

I, _____, agree to _____
        (child's name)

_____

_____

_____

_____.

We, Mom and Dad, agree to _____

_____

_____

_____

_____.

Date contract begins: _____

Date contract is reevaluated: _____

Date contract ends or is renegotiated: _____

_____   _____
Child's Signature   Date

_____   _____
Mother's Signature   Date

_____   _____
Dad's Signature   Date

Menu of Rewards

Menu of Privileges and Rewards	Cost in Points/Chips
1.	
2.	
3.	
4.	
5.	
6.	
7.	
8.	
9.	
10.	

Weekly Point Chart

Behavior (points)	Mon.	Tues.	Wed.	Thurs.	Fri.	Sat.	Sun.
1) ( )							
2) ( )							
3) ( )							
4) ( )							
5) ( )							
6) ( )							
Total points earned							

Child's Signature   Date   Mother's Signature   Date

Father's Signature   Date

Directions:
Each time a behavior is checked, award the points earned and praise the child. Total the points at the end of each day. Draw marks through the points when the child spends them on a reward. Begin a new chart each week.

Problem-Solving Worksheet

1. **S**TOP: What is the problem? _____

   _____

2. **T**HINK of as many plans as possible that might help to solve the problem.

   _____   _____

   _____   _____

   _____   _____

3. **P**ICK the best plan.

   _____

   _____

   _____

   _____

   _____

   _____

4. **D**O the plan.

5. **E**VALUATE the plan. Was it a good plan? _____ Yes _____ No

   How did it work?

   _____

   _____

   _____

   _____

School Monitoring Card

Name: _____ Date: _____

Behavior	7:30–9:00	9:00–10:30	10:30–12:30	12:30–2:30
1.				
2.				
3.				

_____   _____   _____
Parent's Signature   Child's Signature   Teacher's Signature

Weekly Goal Contract

This week's goals are the following:

1. _____

2. _____

3. _____

If _____
        Student's Name

reaches the goals,

_____

_____ .
                                    Reward

If _____
        Student's Name

does *not* reach the goals,

_____

_____ .
                                 Consequence

_____   _____
Student's Signature   Date   Coach's Signature   Date

_____   _____
Parent's Signature   Date   Parent's Signature   Date

References

Abramowitz, A. J., & O'Leary, S. G. (1991). Behavioral interventions for the classroom: Implications for students with ADHD. *School Psychology Review, 20,* 220–234.

American Psychiatric Association. (1994). *Diagnostic and statistical manual of mental disorders* (4th ed.). Washington, DC: Author.

Ames, L. B., Ilg, F. L., & Baker, S. M. (1988). *Your ten to fourteen-year-old.* New York: Delta.

Archer, A., & Gleason, M. (1989). *Skills for school success.* North Billerica, MA: Curriculum Associates.

Bachman, J., Green, S., & Wirtanen, I. (1971). *Dropping out—Problem or symptom?* Vol. 3, *Youth in transition.* Ann Arbor, MI: Institute for Social Research, University of Michigan.

Baker, L., & Cantwell, D. P. (1977). Psychiatric disorder in children with speech and language retardation. *Archives of General Psychiatry, 34,* 583–591.

Baldwin, B. (1988). *Beyond the cornucopia kids.* Wilmington, NC: Direction Dynamics.

Barkley, R. A. (1995). *Taking charge of ADHD.* New York: Guilford Press.

Bosco, J., & Robin, S. (1980). Hyperkinesis: Prevalence and treatment. In C. Whalen & B. Henker (Eds.), *Hyperactive children: The social ecology of identification and treatment* (pp. 173–187). New York: Academic Press.

Briggs, D. C. (1975). *Your child's self-esteem: The key to life.* Garden City, NY: Doubleday.

Brink, C. R. (1972). *The bad times of Irma Bawnlein.* Old Tappan, NJ: Simon & Schuster.

Brooks, R. B. (1991). *The self-esteem teacher.* Circle Pines, MN: American Guidance Service.

Brooks, R. B. (1992). Self-esteem during the school years, its normal development and hazardous decline. *Development and Behavior: Older Children and Adolescents, 39,* 537–550.

Canfield, J., & Hansen, M. V. (1995). *A 2nd Helping of Chicken Soup for the Soul.* Deerfield Beach, FL: Health Communications, Inc.

Carlson, C. L., Pelham, W. E., Milich, R., & Dixon, J. (1992). Single and combined effects of methylphenidate and behavior therapy on the classroom performance of children with attention deficit hyperactivity disorder. *Journal of Abnormal Child Psychology, 20,* 213–232.

Chess, S., & Thomas, A. (1987). *Know your child.* New York: Basic Books, Inc.

Clark, L. (1989). *The time-out solution: A parent's guide for handling everyday behavior problems.* New York: Comtemporary Books.

Comings, D. E. (1996, October). *Tourette syndrome.* A presentation at the Sixth Annual Ch.A.D.D. Conference, New York.

Conger, J. J. (1977). *Adolescence and youth: Psychological development in a changing world.* New York: Harper.

Curran, D. (1983). *Traits of a healthy family.* New York: Ballantine Books.

Davis, L., Sirotowitz, S., & Parker, H. (1996). *Study strategies made easy: A practical plan for school success.* Plantation, FL: Specialty Press.

Dodson, F. (1978). *How to discipline with love.* New York: New American Library.

Douglas, V. I., Barr, R. G., Amin, K., O'Neill, M. E., & Britton, B. G. (1988). Dosage effects and individual responsivity to methylphenidate in attention deficit disorder. *Journal of Child Psychology and Psychiatry, 29,* 453–475.

Elia, J., Borcherding, B. G., Rapoport, J. L., & Kayser, C. S. (1991). Methylphenidate and dextroamphetamine treatment of hyperactives: Are there true non-responders? *Psychiatry Research, 36,* 141–155.

Engstrom, T. W. (1982). *The pursuit of excellence.* Grand Rapids, MI: Zondervan.

Forgatch, M., & Patterson, G. (1989). *Living together Part 2: Family problem solving.* Eugene, OR: Castalia.

Goldstein, S. (1993, June). ADHD in the adolescent years. *Ch.A.D.D.ER Box, 6*(1), 7–8.

Gordon, M. (1992). *My brother's a world class pain: A sibling's guide to ADHD/hyperactivity.* Dewitt, NY: GSI.

Guevremont, D., Dupaul, G. J., & Barkley, R. A. (1990). Diagnosis and assessment of attention deficit hyperactivity disorder in children. *Journal of School Psychology, 28,* 51–78.

Halpern, A. S. (1994). The transition of youth with disabilities to adult life: A position statement of the Division on Career Development and Transition, the Council for Exceptional Children. *Career Development for Exceptional Individuals, 17,* 115–124.

Hamaguchi, P. (1995). *Childhood speech, language, and listening problems: What every parent should know.* New York: John Wiley and Sons.

Hannah, J. N., & Stafford, D. (1993). *Single parenting with Dick and Jane.* Nashville, TN: Family Touch Press.

Hinshaw, S. P. (1996). Enhancing social competence: Integrating self-management strategies with behavioral procedures for children with ADHD. In E. D. Hibbs & P. S. Jensen (Eds.). *Psychosocial treatments for child and adolescent disorders* (pp. 285–309). Washington, DC: American Psychological Association.

Hinshaw, S. P., Buhrmester, D., & Helleer, T. (1989). Anger control in response to verbal provocation: Effects of stimulant medication for boys with

ADHD. *Journal of Abnormal Child Psychology*, 12, 55–71.

Hinshaw, S. P., Henker, B., Whalen, C. K., Erhardt, D., & Dunnington, R. E. (1989). Aggressive, prosocial, and nonsocial behavior in hyperactive boys: Dose effects of methylphenidate in naturalistic settings. *Journal of Consulting and Clinical Psychology*, 57, 636–643.

Hunt, R., Capper, L., & O'Connell, P. (1990). Clonidine in child and adolescent psychiatry. *Journal of Child and Adolescent Psychopharmacology*, 1, 87–102.

Individuals with Disabilities Education Act of 1990, 20 U.S.C. § 1400 *et seq.*

Jensen, J. B., & Garfinkel, B. D. (1988). Neuroendocrine aspects of attention deficit hyperactivity disorders. *Neurologic Clinics*, 6, 111–129.

Jenson, W. R. (1995, October). *A parent's guide to raising tough kids: A practical parent training approach.* Lecture presented at the Seventh Annual Conference for Ch.A.D.D., Washington, DC.

Kajander, R. (1995). *Living with ADHD: A practical guide to coping with attention deficit hyperactivity disorder.* Minneapolis, MN: Park Nicollet Medical Foundation.

Kehle, R. J., Clark, E., & Jenson, W. R. (1996). Interventions for students with traumatic brain injury: Managing behavioral disturbances. *Journal of Learning Disabilities*, 29, 633–642.

Kersey, K. C. (1987). *The art of sensitive parenting: The 10 master keys to raising confident, competent, and responsible children.* Washington, DC: Acropolis.

Loomans, D., & Loomans, J. (1994). *Full Esteem Ahead.* Tiburon, CA: H. J. Kramer.

Love, A. J., & Thompson, M. G. G. (1988). Language disorders and attention deficit disorder in young children referred for psychiatric services: Analysis of prevalence and a conceptual synthesis. *American Journal of Orthopsychology*, 58, 52–64.

McLaughlin, J. (1995). *Celebrating the positives.* Presentation given to parents in Vanderbilt's Summer Day Treatment Program. Unpublished.

Ness, E. M. (1966). *Sam, Bangs, and Moonshine.* New York: Holt, Rinehart, and Winston.

Patterson, G. R. (1975). *Families: Applications of social learning to family life.* Champaign, IL: Research Press.

Patterson, G. R., & Forgatch, M. (1987). *Parents and adolescents living together* Part 1: *The basics.* Eugene, OR: Castalia.

Pelham, W. E. (1989). Behavior therapy, behavioral assessment, and psychostimulant medication in treatment of attention deficit disorders: An interactive approach. In J. Swanson & L. Bloomingdale (Eds.). *Attention deficit disorders IV: Current concepts and emerging trends in attentional and behavioral disorders of childhood* (pp. 169–195). London: Pergamon.

Pelham, W. E. (1995, October). *School and child based treatment.* Paper presented at the conference for Practical Management of ADHD Children to Young Adults, Palm Beach, FL.

Pennington, B. F. (1991). *Diagnosing learning disorders.* New York: Guilford Press.

Phelan, T. W. (1984). *1-2-3 magic! Training your preschoolers and preteens to do what you want.* Plantation, FL: Child Management.

Pisterman, S., Firestone, P., McGrath, P., Goodman, J. T., Webster, I., Mallory, R., & Goffin, B. (1992). The effects of parent training on parenting stress and sense of competence. *Canadian Journal of Behavioral Science*, 24, 41–58.

Reavis, H. K., Jenson, W. R., Kukic, S. J., & Morgan, D. P. (1993). *Utah's BEST project: Behavioral and educational strategies for teachers.* Salt Lake City: Utah State Office of Education.

Rehabilitation Act of 1973, 29 U.S.C. § 701 *et seq.*

Reid, M. K., & Borkowski, J. G. (1987). Causal attributions of hyperactive children: Implication for teaching strategies and self-control. *Journal of Applied Behavior Analysis*, 9, 335–354.

Robin, A. L., & Foster, S. L. (1989). *Negotiating parent-adolescent conflict: A behavioral-family systems approach.* New York: Guilford Press.

Roderick, M. (1995). Grade retention and school dropout: Policy debate and research questions. *Phi Delta Kappa Research Bulletin*, 15, 1–4.

Ross, D. M., & Ross, S. A. (1976). *Hyperactivity: Research, theory, and action.* New York: John Wiley and Sons.

Schaefer, C. E., & Millman, H. L. (1981). *How to help children with common problems.* New York: Signett.

Sloan, H. N. (1979). *The good kid book: How to solve the 15 most common behavior problems.* Champaign, IL: Research Press.

Steinberg, L., & Levine, A. (1990). *You and your adolescent: A parent's guide for ages 10–20.* New York: Harper Perennial.

Wehman, P. (1995). *Individual transition plans: The teacher's curriculum guide for helping youth with special needs.* Austin, TX: PRO-ED.

Weis, G., & Hechtman, L. T. (1986). *Hyperactive children grown up.* New York: Guilford Press.

Wolraich, M. L., Hannah, J. N., Pinnock, T. Y., Baumgaertel, A., & Brown, J. (1996). Comparison of diagnostic criteria for attention deficit hyperactivity disorder in a county-wide sample. *Journal of Child and Adolescent Psychiatry*, 35, 319–324.

Zentall, S. S., & Gohs, D. E. (1984). Hyperactive and comparison children's response to detailed vs. global cues in communication tasks. *Learning Disability Quarterly*, 7, 77–87.

Zentall, S. S., & Meyer, M. J. (1987). Self-regulation of stimulation for ADD-H children during reading and vigilance task performance. *Journal of Abnormal Child Psychology*, 15, 519–536.

About the Author

Jane N. Hannah, EdD, is an assistant professor of pediatrics at the Child Development Center at the Vanderbilt University Medical Center. Dr. Hannah earned her EdD degree from Peabody of Vanderbilt University and her BS and MEd degrees from Middle Tennessee State University. She is an educational and behavioral specialist who directs the Summer Day Treatment Program (STP) for children with an attention-deficit/hyperactivity disorder and is also supervisor of educational services at Vanderbilt's Child Development Center (CDC). She is a former classroom and special education teacher as well as a supervisor of special education in a Tennessee school system. In addition to having administrative responsibilities at the CDC, she is part of an interdisciplinary team that evaluates children who have learning and/or behavioral problems.

Dr. Hannah works extensively with parents of children with behavior problems and consults with teachers and other professionals in developing appropriate educational and/or behavioral plans for children with educational, social, or behavioral problems. She has led parent groups for the past eight years. She is a charter member of the Tennessee chapter of the Council for Learning Disabilities (CLD) and a past president of TCLD, is currently on the Board of Tennessee chapter, and was a local co-arrangements chair of the 18th International Conference on Learning Disabilities held in Nashville, Tennessee, in 1996.

Dr. Hannah is married to Larry Pendergrass, and she has three children and two stepchildren. Her children are Julie Hannah Allen, G. Thomas Hannah Jr., and Emily Elizabeth Hannah. Her stepchildren are Dolly and Mancy Pendergrass. Julie is a business development associate with Star Bank in Bowling Green, Kentucky; Thomas is a constuction foreman with Mark Poe Construction Company in Nashville, Tennessee; Emily is a senior at the University of Kentucky; Dolly is a senior at Belmont University in Nashville; and Mancy is a musician in Franklin, Tennessee. Her husband, Larry, is a sales representative with ALT Communications in Nashville.